Springer
Tokyo
Berlin
Heidelberg
New York
Barcelona
Hong Kong
London
Milan
Paris
Singapore

Recent Advances in Endourology, 3

M. Akimoto, E. Higashihara
H. Kumon, Z. Masaki, S. Orikasa (Eds.)

Treatment of Urolithiasis

With 43 Figures, Including 1 in Color

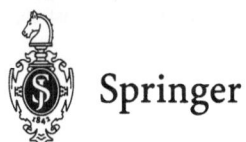

Springer

Masao Akimoto, M.D.
Professor and Chairman, Department of Urology, Nippon Medical School, 1-1-5 Sendagi,
Bunkyo-ku, Tokyo 113-8603, Japan

Eiji Higashihara, M.D.
Professor, Department of Urology, Kyorin University, 6-20-2 Shinkawa, Mitaka, Tokyo 181-
8611, Japan

Hiromi Kumon, M.D.
Professor, Department of Urology, Okayama University Graduate School of Medicine and
Dentistry, 2-5-1 Shikata-cho, Okayama 700-8558, Japan

Zenjiro Masaki, M.D.
Professor, Department of Urology, Saga Medical School, 5-1-1 Nabeshima, Saga 849-8501, Japan

Seiichi Orikasa, M.D.
Professor, Department of Urology, Tohoku University, 1-1 Seiryo-machi, Aoba-ku, Sendai 980-
8574, Japan

ISBN-13: 978-4-431-68519-7

Library of Congress Cataloging-in-Publication Data

Treatment of urolithiasis / M. Akimoto . . . [et al.], (eds.).
    p. ; cm. — (Recent advances in endourology ; 3)
    Includes bibliographical references and index.
    ISBN-13: 978-4-431-68519-7   e-ISBN-13: 978-4-431-68517-3
    DOI: 10.1007/978-4-431-68517-3

    1. Urinary organs—Calculi—Treatment. 2. Extracorporeal shock wave lithotripsy. I.
Akimoto, Masao, 1935– II. Series.
    [DNLM: 1. Urinary Calculi—therapy. 2. Lithotripsy. WJ 100 T784 2001]
    RC916.T74 2001
    616.6'2206—dc21

                                                                    2001032081

Printed on acid-free paper

Typesetting: Best-set Typesetter Ltd., Hong Kong

SPIN: 10833358 series number 4130

Preface

Urolithiasis is not only one of the most frequently encountered diseases at urological clinics; it is also the disorder whose treatment has shown the most rapid progress in the past decade. In that period, medicine has experienced a real revolution, characterized by minimally invasive treatments, improvement of the quality of life, and cost-effectiveness in treatment outcomes. In urology, the revolution started with the development of endoscopic retrograde treatment of urolithiasis in the upper urinary tract, which led to development of the percutaneous antegrade maneuver in the latter half of the 1970s. The most remarkable event occurred in 1982, when clinical use of extracorporeal shock wave lithotripsy was introduced by the Munich group, represented by Dr. Christian Chaussy, at the 18th Congress of the International Society of Urology in San Francisco. With the advent of these new strategies, open surgery for urolithiasis has all but disappeared. Today, with the availability of new technology and equipment, guidelines for the treatment of urolithiasis have changed in all developed countries. It is quite timely that the Meeting of International Consultation on Urolithiasis will be held in Paris in June 2001 to establish international guidelines for urolithiasis.

Looking through this textbook for urolithiasis, I was greatly impressed to learn that we have already drawn up some guidelines. The book includes all the updated advances of urolithiasis presented by the most prominent and experienced urologists from all around the world. I am quite confident that a great benefit will be assured not only for those who are new to the field but also for specialists, in obtaining the latest knowledge of urolithiasis and treatment techniques.

March 2001
YOSHIO ASO, M.D.
Honorary President, JSEE
Immediate Past President, SIU
Professor Emeritus, The University of Tokyo

Contents

Contributors

Clinical Practice Guidelines for Ureteral Stones: Implications in Japan and Limitations

EIJI HIGASHIHARA

Historical and Social Background of the Development of Clinical Practice Guidelines

Owing to the development of systematic and structured abstraction methods, evidence-based guidelines have been proposed in many disciplines, mainly in the United States of America [1]. A social background which forces practitioners to draw up clinical guidelines is especially strong in the USA, where the medical supply system is exposed to a market economy. The problem of escalating medical costs in the USA prompted the government and the medical insurance companies to introduce clinical practice guidelines. These guidelines were introduced to control medical costs and quality, because many studies had shown wide variations in physician practice patterns and the use of the health services [1]. The health services are used inappropriately in some cases, and the health outcome is made uncertain by the use or nonuse of the various services and procedures. Initially, it was mainly the users of the services who began to develop guidelines, but professionals soon recognized the importance of clinical practice guidelines. The involvement of diverse groups in guidelines development has intensified the need to create and improve scientific methods to develop these guidelines, otherwise they will not be accepted by all groups whatever their economic interests and attitudes.

Purpose of Guidelines

The purpose of clinical guidelines is to standardize treatment outcomes and the costs of treatment. The treatment procedures selected for a particular disease and its expected outcome vary among physicians, and these variances should be minimized by using clinical guidelines. The process of minimizing these variations not

Department of Urology, Kyorin University School of Medicine, 6-20-2 Shinkawa, Mitaka, Tokyo 181-8611, Japan only reduces the range of distribution, but also improves the average level of treatment outcomes, because the groups in which the best possible outcome is already achieved will not generally be affected.

The guidelines are basically a summary of published treatments with statistical analyses of their clinical outcomes. The method used to summarize the outcome of different treatment procedures is statistical metaanalysis. Therefore, the results inevitably depend on published findings. Metaanalysis is limited by the source of information rather than by the methods used.

Science-based guidelines serve to improve the quality of clinical care and its measurement, and to reduce the financial costs of inappropriate care. The major purposes of guidelines are (1) assisting clinical decision-making by patients and practitioners, (2) educating individuals or groups, (3) assessing and ensuring the quality of care, (4) guiding the distribution of resources for health care, and (5) reducing the risk of legal liability for careless treatment [2]. The potential benefits of guidelines are diverse, and the guidelines are not necessarily synonymous with the coverage policies of health insurance plans. The conflict between the person who pays, the consumer, and the practitioner cannot be resolved by having guidelines, but guidelines are rational social judgments about what care should be covered by public and private health benefit plans.

Clinical practice guidelines should be constructed systematically and based on good science practice, and structured abstracting methods were developed for this purpose. In this sense, the scientific guidelines differ from the older type of guidelines proposed by professional organizations or individuals. Many of the guidelines and recommendations found in older literature and textbooks adopted methods which were very different from evidence-based abstraction. Although scientific abstraction methods have now been introduced, there remain significant gaps between what is needed and what is known. These gaps are usually covered by the opinions of leading professionals or their peer group. However, these opinions are rarely based on evidence; and should be replaced by guidelines based on future findings.

Background of the Development of Guidelines in Japan

In Japan, the medical insurance and reimbursement system is tightly controlled by the government, and is not directly exposed to the market economy. The clinical practice reimbursement guidelines (CPRGs) booklet and local reimbursement judgment committees regulate the reimbursement of medical costs. CPRGs are decided solely by the government (Department of Health, Welfare, and Labor). The Japanese Medical Association and other professional medical groups in Japan cannot directly participate in the construction of CPRGs. The CPRGs booklet is renewed yearly from an economic standpoint, and taking into account medical appropriateness. The framework of the CPRGs is limited by supply-side (Government) economics. Hence, the quality of hospital management and medical care are regulated by budget limitations. The consumer-side needs (patients' needs) are of secondary importance. In contrast to the USA, the policymaker's involvement in Japan is negligible, and is regarded as being related to their private interests.

In the Japanese system, a local reimbursement judgment committee checks the expenditures of individual medical practices. The reimbursement is refused if the committee regards the expenditure as inappropriate. The application standards of the local reimbursement judgment committee are based on the CPRGs. The problems are two-fold. The application standard, i.e., the interpretation of the CPRGs, differs from committee to committee and from member to member of the committee, which may reflect personal preferences. The second problem is the medical limitations of the CPRGs, which do not necessarily keep pace with the progress of clinical medicine or with what is appropriate in clinical practice.

The Japanese health care reimbursement system works outside market principles. Patients receive medical care as required, and people regard medical care as being free. In order to safeguard the people's welfare, the medical supply side is required to supply medical care whenever necessary. The practitioner must provide what the patient needs as long as it is appropriate in terms of the CPRGs. This is the background of unlimited medical sources and escalating medical costs which resulted in the government's tight control of expenditure.

The 21st century will be the era of the market economy, which will penetrate into every social field, including government activities, education, and the medical system. The overwhelming growth of the market economy will widen the differences in economic status between individuals and between countries. The gap between industrialized and developing countries will be increased. The rich people will become richer and poor people will stay poor. A market economy develops energy-consuming industries and harms the Earth's environment. The two greatest negative aspects of the market economy will produce two forces working against its development. Ecological forces and the movement of poor people will modify the penetration of the market economy. If any industries or products satisfy market principles as well as environmental protectionism, that field will expand very rapidly, as experienced recently in industries generating electricity using solar and wind power.

In spite of the difficulties facing the medical care supply system, the government, the people (patients), and clinical practitioners in Japan are reluctant to bring a market economy system even partially into the medical supply system. However, the tightly regulated government system has a limited ability to adapt to the rapid progress occurring in clinical medicine. Therefore, highly developed clinical practices are seen as suitable area to introduce high-technology medicine at the patient's own expense. In this system, the introduction of a new clinical practice into an institution is allowed after an evaluation of its appropriateness. The patient covers the medical costs of the new practice, while all related medical expenditure is covered by the medical insurance system. The combination of personal payment and a social insurance system makes the medical supply system flexible. This combination will develop further in circumstances of budgetary restraint.

Implications of the Introduction of Clinical Practice Guidelines in Japan

The social and economic significance of clinical guidelines in Japan differ from those in the USA. As mentioned above, medical practice guidelines are already operational in Japan. Since the CPRG system was introduced in 1963, no clinical practice has been covered if it violates the guidelines. The CPRG system is applied more strictly year by year, and clinical practice is regulated by the CPRG system. Consequently, the inappropriate use of clinical practices is limited. However, new techniques with high-quality health outcomes, such as laparoscopy, preventive medicine, and quality of living-related medicine, are inevitably restricted.

The problem with the CPRG system is the principle used to develop the guidelines. This is not an evidence-based scientific approach, but is a bureaucrat's opinion taken from the standpoint of the budget or the prevention of inappropriate use of medical care. Professionals and medical groups express their opinions about the content of the CPRGs, but these are generally ignored. Clinical practice guidelines are not synonymous with the reimbursement or coverage policies of the CPRGs system, and the two should not be confused. However, if science-based clinical guidelines are introduced into Japan by professionals, and clinical practices are still performed in a guideline-compatible manner, then problems will arise. The introduction of guidelines did help to correct the wide variations in physician practice patterns, and did reduce the inappropriate use of many services. At present many clinical techniques which science-based guidelines would allow are restricted by the CPRGs system. The incompatibility between science-based clinical practice guidelines and the CPRGs system is becoming a problem. Another problem which arises from the introduction of clinical guidelines is the resistance of clinical practitioners and health-related groups. Private practitioners do not like tight controls. The CPRGs system is not only handling reimbursements or coverage policies, but has already extended its role into the work of practitioners. The CPRGs system needs to be reconstructed in a manner which is compatible with science-based guidelines.

Clinical Practice Guidelines for Ureteral Stones

As the result of an enormous effort by the members of the American Urological Association (AUA), clinical guidelines for ureteral stones have recently been proposed [2, 3]. The structure of these guidelines is new, and their theme covers major clinical entities such as benign prostatic hypertrophy, incontinence, and urolithiasis. Some differences of opinion and/or cases of insufficient evidence which appear in the "Clinical Practice Guidelines for Ureteral Stones" of the AUA [2] are discussed below.

The three main factors which affect the outcome of an evaluation are (1) the definitions of the nature of a stone, (2) methods of evaluating the outcome, and (3) changes in expectations as the result of technological progress.

In addition to treatment modalities and the physician's experience, some factors which affect the outcome of treatment for ureteral stones are the location, size, impaction, and composition of the stone. These factors are discussed below.

Ureteric Divisions

With regard to stone location, the ureter is usually divided into two [2] or three [4–10] portions from the view point of treatment practice. There is no agreement about whether two or three divisions are the most appropriate. Three ureteric divisions, i.e., the upper, middle, and lower thirds of the ureter, have been used in many studies [4–11]. The middle portion corresponds to the segment that overlaps the sacral bone, and the lower portion is the juxtavesical portion of the ureter lying below the iliac bone [10, 12]. For two divisions, the ureter segment is divided into the proximal and distal ureter [2]. The proximal ureter is the segment above the iliac vessels, and includes the upper and middle thirds of the three ureteric divisions (Fig. 1).

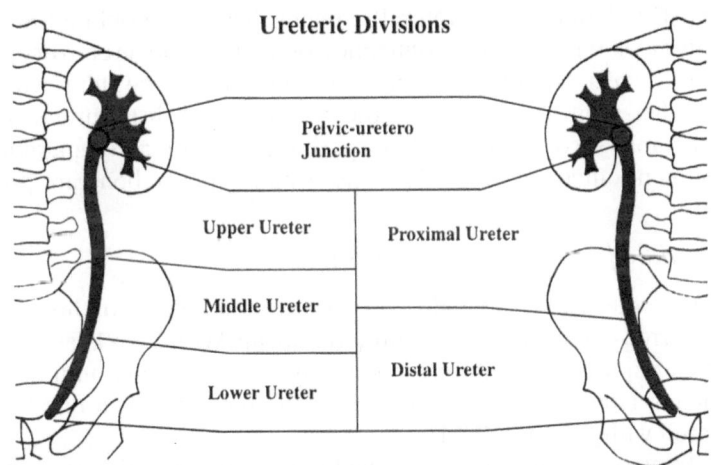

FIG. 1. With two ureteric divisions, the ureter is divided at the point where the ureter crosses the iliac vessels. In a plain X-ray, it is difficult to locate this point precisely. It is clearer if the distal ureter is defined as the ureteral segment below the upper pelvic rim, which includes the middle and lower ureteric segments in the three-division system. Two divisions may be adequate from the standpoint of ureteroscopic treatment, but three divisions are more practical from the standpoint of ESWL treatment of ureteral stones

From the standpoint of ureteroscopy, the proximal and distal divisions are sufficient. Stones in the distal segment are easily accessible using a rigid ureteroscope. Using an actively deflectable flexible ureteroscope for proximal ureteral stones gives a much better outcome than a rigid one, which leads to a small difference in the treatment outcomes between the two locations. This simple division of the ureteral segment may be adequate as technology develops, since treatment outcomes do not differ much between the middle and lower segments [4, 5]. Therefore, two divisions appear to be adequate for ureteroscopic treatment of ureteral stones.

The main issue is which point is suitable for the separation of the two divisions. The physiological narrowing of the ureter where it curves over the iliac vessels is not an obstacle for a small-caliber ureteroscope. If the ureter is divided into two segments, the point of division should be the upper brim of the iliac bone, because treatment outcomes are significantly different above and below the pelvic crest [5, 6].

For extracorporeal shockwave lithotripsy (ESWL), three divisions are more practical. The middle ureteral segment overlaps the sacral bone that impedes shockwave penetration. In some shockwave lithotriptors, the ultrasound system is used for stone localization. The pelvic bone is also an obstacle for ultrasound monitoring. Therefore, the ureteral segment that overlaps the pelvic bone has a significant meaning for shockwave treatment [10, 12].

The treatment of ureteral stones is mostly by ESWL and ureteroscopy, and less frequently by percutaneous nephrolithotomy, retroperitoneoscopy, or open surgery. The definition of ureteral segment divisions should allow an adequate evaluation of the treatment outcomes of ESWL and ureteroscopy. However, the iliac vessels cannot be distinguished by plain X-ray film, which results in a somewhat arbitrary division of the proximal and distal ureter. For easy and demonstrable recognition of stone position, and for a comparable evaluation of treatment outcomes, three divisions using the pelvic bone are preferable.

Methods of Outcome Evaluation

Recently, either ESWL or endoscopic transurethral ureterolithotripsy have been the preferred choice for treating ureteral calculi. With ESWL, auxiliary measures are often required, and multiple sessions may be necessary until the treatment is completed. However, the invasiveness of ureteroscopy is a disadvantage when compared with ESWL [10, 11].

The treatment outcomes are evaluated from the resulting stone-free rate, the number of treatments including the auxiliary procedures, the invasiveness of the treatment, and complications or other morbidities associated with the treatment. The evaluation of treatment methods for ureteral stones might be improved by summing up these factors, but an integrated method to achieve this does not yet exist. In general, the stone-free rate is selected as the most important determining factor [4–10]. The complication rate and other factors are considered to be of secondary importance and are analyzed separately. This separate analysis of factors other than stone-free rate tends to obscure outcome evaluations of treatment modalities. The treatment options recommended by the clinical guidelines are only loosely defines owing to the many analytical methods reported [2]. For any comparison of treatment modalities, it is necessary to weigh these factors appropriately.

Clayman et al. [13] introduced an effectiveness quotient to compare the various extracorporeal shock wave lithotripters available. The quotient for ESWL is

$$\frac{\% \text{ Stone free}}{100\% + \% \text{ Re-treatment} + \% \text{ Auxiliary procedures}} \times 100$$

This quotient was developed in order to compare the effectiveness of lithotripters used in previously reported studies. However, this quotient design has limitations, and it is not possible for the difference between two or more lithotripters to be clarified statistically [10, 11, 13].

The equation used to formulate a treatment effectiveness and quality (TEQ) score is shown in Fig. 2. The TEQ score was developed from the effectiveness quotient. The TEQ score compares the treatment modalities based on individual findings or measurements, and thus is able to clarify the difference statistically. The equation considers not only the stone-free rate, but also the number of auxiliary measures, the invasiveness of the treatment modality, and any complications in an integrated manner.

The coefficients of the TEQ score were chosen arbitrarily, and no set of coefficients has a concrete meaning. This limitation can be overcome by large

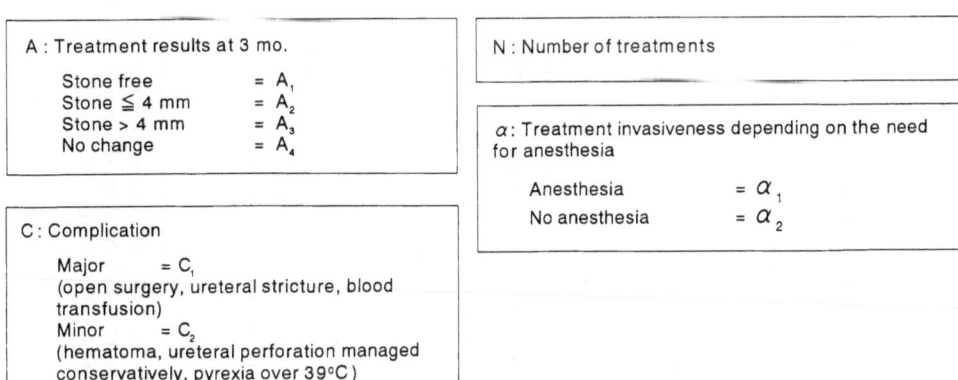

$$\text{TEQ Score} = \frac{A - C}{\Sigma \alpha_i N_i}$$

| A : Treatment results at 3 mo. | N : Number of treatments |

A : Treatment results at 3 mo.

Stone free   = A_1
Stone $\leq$ 4 mm   = A_2
Stone > 4 mm   = A_3
No change   = A_4

N : Number of treatments

α : Treatment invasiveness depending on the need for anesthesia

Anesthesia   = α_1
No anesthesia   = α_2

C : Complication

Major   = C_1
(open surgery, ureteral stricture, blood transfusion)
Minor   = C_2
(hematoma, ureteral perforation managed conservatively, pyrexia over 39°C)

FIG. 2. TEQ scores are calculated using the formula shown and assigning the appropriate numbers, e.g., $A_1 = 100$, $A_2 = 75$,..., $C_1 = 100$, $C_2 = 50$, $\alpha_1 = 1$, and $\alpha_2 = 0.8$

TABLE 1. Results of ureteral stone treatment by ureteroscopy

Authors	Year	Ref. No	Outer diameter of ureteroscope	Lithotriptor	No. of cases	Success rate (%)	Uret. perf. or strict.	Open surgery
Group 1								
Lingeman et al.	1986	15	11–14 Fr./rigid	US, EHL	147	83	16	3
Tanahashi et al.	1986	16	11–14 Fr./rigid	US, EHL	121	74	1	1
Ono et al.	1987	17	11–14 Fr./rigid	US, EHL	122	76	12	3
Weiberg et al.	1987	18	11–14 Fr./rigid	US	127	82	3	1
Total					511	79	32 (6.3%)	8 (1.6%)
Group 2								
Govier et al.	1990	19	9.5 Fr./rigid	Pulsed-dye	50	88	1	1
Fugelso and Neal	1991	20	7.2 Fr./rigid	Pulsed-dye	204	97	5	0
Vorreuther	1992	21	6.5 Fr./rigid	EHL	85	91	1	0
Van Deursen et al.	1991	22	7.5 Fr./rigid	Pulsed-dye	204	90	2	0
Total					543	93	9 (1.7%)	1 (0.2%)
P-value group 1 vs. 2						<.01	<.01	<.05
Group 3								
Murthy et al.	1997	23	7.2 Fr./semirigid	Lithoclast	122	97.3	0	0
Gould	1998	24	7.2 Fr./semirigid	Ho:YAG laser	127	96.9	0	0
Grasso and Bagley	1998	25	$\leqq$8 Fr./flexible	Ho:YAG laser	122	97	0.5	0
Tawfick and Bagley	1999	26	7.5–9.8 Fr./SR/flexible	Ho:YAG laser	82	98.8	0	0
Total					453	97	0.5 (0.1%)	0 (0%)
P-value group 2 vs. 3						<.01	<.05	NS

Uret. perf. or strict., number of cases of ureteral perforation or stricture; SR, semirigid.
The success rate equals the stone-free rate in group 3.
P-values were obtained by the χ^2 test.

alterations in the variables. The TEQ score will change as the variables change, and these changes will indicate which score is better.

Size of Stones and Stone Impaction

Stone size is an important factor affecting treatment outcomes, and usually, stratification is at a stone size of 10 mm in diameter on X-rays [2, 5]. It is recognized that impacted stones resist ESWL treatment [7, 8, 14]. However, a definition of an impacted stone has not yet been established, and it is not known whether stone size or stone impaction has the greater effect on treatment outcomes. An impacted stone is usually defined as one where impaction has been confirmed by ureteroscopy, or where it is not possible to pass a ureteral stent beyond the stone [7, 8, 14]. However, impacted stones must be identified before ureteroscopy, otherwise treatment outcomes between ESWL and ureteroscopic treatment cannot be compared. The following three criteria are suggested as a definition of stone impaction: (1) unchanged stone location for at least 1 month; (2) no severe pain for at least 3 months; (3) the existence of hydronephrosis to any degree. These criteria are applicable to any ureteral stone before any treatment.

Time Effect on Treatment Outcome

The development of ureteroscopes (small-caliber, flexible, actively deflectable, and with large working channels), lithotriptors (effective stone disintegration, less harmful, adaptable to a small working channel), and other techniques all contribute to better treatment outcomes and lower complication rates, as shown in Table 1. The treatment results are divided into three groups based on the year of publication. The publication date differs by about 5 years between the three groups. The caliber of ureteroscopes was smaller in group 2 than in group 1, and the better outcomes might be the result of the miniaturized scope. However, treatment outcomes were further improved in group 3, despite no further miniaturization of the scopes. A smaller diameter is certainly less harmful to the ureter and eases access to the urinary tract, but a wide working channel is required for the smooth manipulation of lithotriptors and various forceps. The outer diameters of the fiber of pulsed-dye lasers and holmium:YAG lasers are around 300–1000 μm, a size which is adequate for a ureteroscope. Therefore, a 6–7 Fr. ureteroscope is appropriate at the present technological level of manufacture.

Improvements in the treatment outcomes between groups 2 and 3 were not due to smaller caliber ureteroscopes, but to improvements in the lithotriptors and the learning curve of endoscopists. These improvements in outcome require periodic revision of the practice guidelines.

References

1. Field MJ, Lohr KN (1992) Guidelines for clinical practice. National Academy Press, Washington, DC

2. Segura JW, Preminger GM, Assimos DG, Dretler SP, Kahn RI, Lingeman JE. Macaluso JN (1997) Report on the management of ureteral calculi. The American Urological Association Ureteral Stones Clinical Guidelines Panel
3. Segura JW, Assimos DG, Dretler SP, Kahn RI, Lingeman JE, Preminger GM. Macaluso JN, McCullough DL, Roehrborn CG (1994) Report on the management of staghorn calculi. The American Urological Association Ureteral Stones Clinical Guidelines Panel
4. Bierkens AF, Hendrikx AJM, De La Rosette JJMCH, Stultiens GNM, Beerlage HP, Arends AJ, Debruyne FMJ (1998) Treatment of mid and lower ureteric calculi: extracorporeal shock-wave lithotripsy vs. laser ureteroscopy. A comparison of costs, morbidity and effectiveness. Br J Urol 81:31–35
5. Park H, Park M, Park T (1998) Two-year experience with ureteral stones: extracorporeal shockwave lithotripsy v. ureteroscopic manipulation. J Endourol 12:501–504
6. Osti AH, Hofmockel G, Frohmuller H (1997) Ureteroscopic treatment of ureteral stones: only an auxiliary measure of extracorporeal shockwave lithotripsy or a primary therapeutic option? Urol Int 59:177–181
7. Dretler SP, Keating MA, Riley J (1986) An algorithm for the management of ureteral calculi. J Urol 136:1190–1193
8. Morgentaler A, Bridge SS, Dretler SP (1990) Management of the impacted ureteral calculus. J Urol 143:263–266
9. Roberts WW, Cadeddu JA, Micali S, Kavoussi LR (1998) Ureteral stricture formation after removal of impacted calculi. J Urol 159:723–726
10. Singal RK, Denstedt JD (1997) Contemporary management of ureteric stones. Urol Clin North Am 24:59–70
11. Hendrikx AJM, Strijbos WEM, de Knijff DW, Kums JJM, Doesburg WH, Lemmens WAJG (1999) Treatment for extended mid and distal ureteral stones: SWL or ureteroscopy? Results of a multicenter study. J Endourol 13:727–733
12. Sonoda T (1989) Assessment guideline for treatment of urolithiasis by endourology and ESWL. Jpn J Urol (Nihon Hinyokika Gakaizashi) 80:505–506
13. Clayman RV, McClennan BL, Garvin TJ, Denstedt JD, Andriole GL (1989) Lithostar: an electromagnetic acoustic shock wave unit for extracorporeal lithotripsy. J Endourol 3:307–313
14. Srivastava A, Ahlawat R, Kumar A, Kapoor R, Bhandari M (1992) Management of impacted upper ureteric calculi: results of lithotripsy and percutaneous litholapaxy. Br J Urol 70:252–257
15. Lingeman JE, Sonda LP, Kahnoski RJ, Coury TA, Newmwn DM, Mosbaugh PG, Mertz JHO, Steele RE, Frank B (1986) Ureteral stone management: emerging concepts. J Urol 135:1172–1174
16. Tanahashi Y, Kuwahara M, Kanbe K, Chiba Y, Kuros S, Kageyama S, Numata I, Orikasa S (1986) Transurethral ureterolithotripsy (first report). Jpn J Urol 77:1082–1088
17. Ono Y, Hirabayashi S, Yamada S, Ohosima S, Kinukawa T, Matuura O, Katoh N, Sugiyma T, Watanabe J (1987) Transurethral lithotripsy: preliminary report. Jpn J Urol 78:1917–1922
18. Weiberg JJ, Ansong K, Smith AD (1987) Complications of ureteroscopy in relation to experience: report of surgery and another experience. J Urol 137:384–385
19. Govier FE, Gibbon RP, Correa RJ, Brannen GE, Welssman RM, Pritchett TR (1990) Pulsed-dye laser fragmentation of ureteral calculi: a review of the first 50 cases performed at Virginia Mason Medical Center. J Urol 143:685–686

20. Fugelso P, Neal PM (1991) Endoscopic laser lithotripsy: safe, effective therapy for ureteral calculi. J Urol 145:949–951
21. Vorreuther R (1992) Minimally invasive ureteroscopy using adjustable electrohydraulic lithotripsy. J Endourol 6:47–50
22. Van Deursen H, Pottomvils G, Boving R, Baert L (1991) Pulsed-dye laser lithotripsy. Which laser fiber is preferable? Critical evaluation in 204 consecutive lasertripsies. J Endurol 5:301–305
23. Murthy PV, Rao HSG, Meherwade S, Rao S, Srivastava A, Sasidharan K (1997) Ureteroscopic lithotripsy using a mini-endoscope and Swiss lithoclast: experience in 147 cases. J Endourol 11:327–330
24. Gould DL (1998) Holmium:YAG laser and its use in the treatment of urolithiasis: our first 160 cases. J Endourol 12:23–26
25. Grasso M, Bagley D (1998) Small-diameter, actively deflectable, flexible ureteropyeloscopy. J Urol 160:1648–1654
26. Tawfiek ER, Bagley D (1999) Management of upper urinary tract calculi with ureteroscopic techniques. Urology 53:25–31

Management of Urolithiasis: Guidelines in the USA

SANJAY RAMAKUMAR[1] and JOSEPH W. SEGURA[2]

Summary. The surgical management of urinary calculi is often varied. Factors such as patient characteristics and the availability of treatment modalities are influential in determining a course of action. In the United States, the approach has been more invasive than in other countries owing to economic and patient factors. Distal ureteral stones are usually treated ureteroscopically, and smaller renal and upper ureteral stones are treated by extracorporeal shockwave lithotripsy (ESWL). Percutaneous lithotripsy is also frequently used for larger renal stones or those which are deemed to have failed ESWL. The practitioner's proficiency in stone extraction techniques also determines the method of treatment. Ultimately, most urinary stones can be treated with minimally invasive techniques.

Key Words. Urolithiasis, ESWL, Ureteroscopy, Percutaneous lithotripsy, Management

Introduction

The surgical management of urinary calculi is often varied. Factors such as patient characteristics and the availability of treatment modalities are influential in determining a course of action. Selecting an option can then become somewhat difficult. Several key points about the American perspective on the management of urolithiasis will be illustrated in this chapter.

[1] Johns Hopkins University, Brady Urological Institute, USA
[2] Department of Urology, Mayo Clinic, 200 1st St. SW, Rochester, MN 55905, USA

Renal Calculi

Although most small renal stones can be treated effectively with shockwave lithotripsy (SWL), the success rate decreases as the stone volume increases. Percutaneous nephrolithotomy (PNL) clearly has advantages in the removal of larger stones with minimal morbidity [1]. This point of transition was generally thought to be 2 cm. Lam et al. [2] performed a more accurate measurement of staghorn stones. By using computer analysis, the stone surface area was measured in patients treated with PNL with or without SWL, and SWL monotherapy. The overall stone-free rate was 84.2% for PNL and 51.2% for SWL. Stones smaller than 500 mm^2 were cleared completely in 63.2% of patients treated with SWL alone. However, in those patients whose stones were smaller than 500 mm^2 and who had a nondilated renal collecting system, the stone-free rate was 91.7%. The use of better selection criteria increased the success of SWL.

Larger lower pole renal calculi do not clear well after SWL, and this is probably a factor of the anatomy the stone fragments must overcome in order to pass. Lingeman et al. [3] have demonstrated, through personal experience and a meta-analysis of the literature, a 90% stone-free rate after PNL, but only a 59% rate after SWL for lower pole stones. Stone-free rates for PNL were independent of stone burden, and were inversely correlated in SWL. Stones in the lower pole less than 2 cm in diameter may be better treated with primary SWL [4]. Elbahnasy et al. [5] have identified the parameters of renal spatial anatomy that influence stone passage. Unfavorable characteristics are an infundibulopelvic angle less than 70°, an infundibular length greater than 3 cm, and an infundibular width less than 5 mm. When all three factors are present, the success of SWL falls to less than 50%. Keeley et al. [6] have found the infundibulopelvic angle to be the most significant factor associated with lower pole stone clearance after SWL.

Staghorn Calculi

Staghorn calculi, or stones that occupy all or most of the collecting system, require careful planning and efficient use of treatment options [7]. The Nephrolithiasis Clinical Guidelines Panel believes that newly diagnosed staghorn calculi should be treated to protect renal function from deterioration [8]. As a guideline, "sandwich therapy" [9], or PNL followed by SWL and repeated PNL, should be used for most patients with standard staghorn calculi. Smaller calculi can be treated with either SWL or PNL when the renal anatomy is normal or near normal. As a general guideline, neither SWL monotherapy nor open surgery should be used as first line of treatment. However, if a stone cannot be managed in a reasonable number of SWL or PNL sessions, open surgery is a reasonable option. Nephrectomy is reserved for poorly functioning stone-bearing kidneys.

In a randomized prospective study, 50 kidneys with complete staghorn calculi were treated with SWL alone ($n = 27$) or PNL with SWL ($n = 23$) [10]. After therapy, the stone-free rate was significantly higher in the PNL group (74% vs. 22%), and the complication rate was greater with SWL alone. There was no significant difference in the number of procedures performed or hospital days, but the number of unplanned ancillary procedures was greater in the SWL monotherapy group. These striking results support the conclusion that complete staghorn calculi should not be treated with SWL alone.

Caliceal Diverticular Calculi

Symptomatic stones in caliceal diverticula are usually treated percutaneously. An ultrasound probe is helpful in fragmenting and removing the stones simultaneously. If the parenchyma overlying the diverticulum is adequate, the neck of the cavity can be dilated and a nephrostomy placed across it until maturity. Diverticula with minimal or absent surrounding parenchyma can be fulgurated, and the nephrostomy tube is used as a perinephric drain. Anterior diverticula cannot be accessed percutaneously because of anatomical considerations, and an open or laparoscopic therapy is required. For the laparoscopic technique, we prefer a transperitoneal approach. The pneumoperitoneum can be accessed with either a Veress needle or the open Hasson technique, and should be maintained at 15–20 mmHg pressure. We use a four-trocar approach by placing the camera in the infraumbilical port and three working ports (usually 10 or 12 mm) located midway between the anterorsuperior iliac spine and the umbilicus, subcostally in the anterior axillary line and subcostally in the midclavicular line [11]. For the pelvic kidney, lower abdominal working ports are used in addition to the infraumbilical camera port [12]. A 6 or 7 Fr external ureteral stent is placed in the renal pelvis to aid in identification of the proximal ureter. To approach a stone-filled caliceal diverticulum, the patient is placed in the modified rotated flank position, approximately 60° from supine. The line of Toldt is incised laterally and the colon is reflected medially. Gerota's fascia is dissected off the kidney and the surface is inspected. The diverticulum can appear as a raised lobular area or a pit in the capsule. If the area is questionable, a gallbladder needle can be used to puncture it and the stone can be palpated with the tip. When there is difficulty in finding the stone, intracorporeal sonography or fluoroscopy can be helpful [13]. Typically, the parenchyma overlying the diverticulum is thin and can be incised with electrocautery scissors. Stone material can be removed from the cavity using graspers and suction. The entire cavity, including the connection with the collecting system, is fulgurated with an electrocautery or argon-beam coagulator, and the diverticulum is marsupialized. Closing the neck of the diverticulum with sutures is difficult and usually not necessary. The defect can either be left open, filled with Gerota's fascia/fat, or filled with a synthetic glue material [14]. A closed suction drain should be placed adjacent to the kidney through one of the working ports and the ureteral catheter left to gravity drainage to prevent urinoma formation. The colon is replaced and the abdomen is exited in the usual fashion.

Ureteral Calculi

There have been several studies comparing the efficacy of SWL and ureteroscopy. In a retrospective, nonrandomized review of the treatment of distal ureteral stones, Anderson et al. [15] found stone-free rates of 96% with the HM3 device, 84% with the Lithostar, and 100% with ureteroscopy. All SWL treatments were performed under sedation and on an outpatient basis. They felt that ureteroscopy was more time consuming, involved routine stent placement, and often required general anesthesia, which lead to more hospitalizations. From a cost standpoint, SWL was slightly more expensive than ureteroscopy, but based on their experience they recommended SWL as the optimal first-line therapy for distal calculi.

Recently, Pearle et al. [16] performed a prospective, randomized trial comparing ureteroscopy and SWL for the treatment of distal ureteral stones. Fifty patients were randomized and were well matched. All patients were stone-free, and neither group had significant complications, although five of the ureteroscopy patients had minor complications. The operative times and the hospital stays were less for SWL, and general anesthesia was used in 68% of the ureteroscopy group but only 20% of the SWL patients. Based on their findings, both modalities were equally effective for the treatment of distal stones, but complications and operative times were higher with ureteroscopy.

In a contemporary retrospective analysis of 1121 patients treated for lower ureteral stones, Biri et al. [17] reported a comparison of ureteroscopy and SWL. The most remarkable difference was seen in the stone-free rate, which was 91.8% in the endourological group and 42.2% for SWL. Complications were a bit higher in the ureteroscopy patients when electrohydraulic intracorporeal lithotripsy was performed. A trend for SWL failure was seen with respect to stone size and composition. In the first SWL session, the stone-free rate for stones of less than 10 mm was 34%, but for stones of 11–20 mm the rate dropped to 15.7%, and for stones larger than 21 mm the stone-free rate was 9.4%. In cases where composition analysis was available, poorer results were seen for SWL of harder stones. The stone-free rates of calcium oxalate monohydrate stones with SWL and intracorporeal devices were 41.9% and 69.9%, respectively. For calcium oxalate dihydrate stones, these rates were 57.2% and 97.2% respectively, and for struvite stones they were 46.6% and 89.8%, respectively. Based on almost 9 years of data, the authors recommend SWL as a first-line therapy only for patients who had stones of less than 10 mm without obstruction or evidence of impaction.

The key to understanding when not to use SWL is to identify which stones will fail the initial therapy. Grasso critically reviewed 121 SWL failures that were referred for endourological management to identify patterns that lead to failure [18]. Patients who had failure to clear fragments had a mean stone diameter of 10.3 mm, and the most common stone types were calcium oxalate monohydrate and brushite. In those patients who had failure to fragment, the mean stone diameter was 12.5 mm and stone composition was primarily calcium oxalate monohydrate. Negative variables for successful fragmentation in ureteral calculi included stone impaction and high-grade obstruction. Second- and third-generation lithotriptors comprised the majority of treatment failures referred for endoscopic management.

We must look not only at the overall stone-free results for a technique, but also at the number of auxiliary procedures, retreatments, postoperative office visits, and imaging studies required before a patient is stone-free. This has significant implications for patients, especially those whose professions do not allow the possibility of failure (e.g., airline pilots). Therapy requiring multiple treatment sessions has significant time and economic repercussions. Grasso et al. [19] reviewed 112 patients treated with either SWL or ureteroscopy to determine which method was more efficacious and cost-effective. The majority of patients were treated in an outpatient setting, and anesthesia requirements were similar. Success was defined as complete clearance of the stone burden in the endoscopy group, and residual asymptomatic 2-mm fragments in the SWL group. Stone-free rates in a single session at 1-month follow-up were 95% and 45% for ureteroscopy and SWL, respectively. At 3 months, rates improved to 97% and 62%, respectively. Retreatments and auxiliary procedures were significantly higher in the SWL group (31% vs. 3%), and the mean number of postoperative visits and imaging studies were also higher for SWL (2.07 vs. 1.13). When comparing outpatient ureteroscopic stone removal to SWL monotherapy, the treatment costs were similar. Retreatment and auxiliary procedures more than doubled the cost of SWL.

Comparing the success of SWL and ureteroscopy between different reports is difficult because of varying definitions of "stone-free" status, and because multiple SWL sessions were sometimes used for stone clearance. The definition of stone-free should be complete fragment removal after ureteroscopy, and fragments smaller than 2mm after single-treatment SWL.

Nowadays, the efficacy of a treatment modality is judged not only by completion of the task, but also by the costs incurred during the treatment. Kapoor et al. [20] found ureteroscopy and SWL to have equal efficacy, but the cost of SWL was 60% higher. Wolf et al. [21] also compared the costs and reported that although initial SWL has a slightly higher cost, the addition of auxiliary/ retreatment procedures significantly increased the costs involved.

We have identified certain clinical parameters that portend SWL failure based on a critical analysis of the literature. SWL is effective for stones in the upper ureter, but we believe there is a distinct advantage in endourological management of distal ureteral stones. Modern ureteroscopy has been improved with the development of smaller endoscopes and advanced lithotriptors (laser, pneumatic), and is truly "minimally invasive" in skilled hands.

Transplanted Kidneys

Urolithiasis in a transplanted kidney is a rare occurrence. The reconstructed anatomy of the transplanted ureter reduces the likelihood of fragments passing after extracorporeal shockwave lithotripsy (ESWL). Percutaneous extraction of stones is a very safe and effective method of stone removal [22–24]. The anterior nature of the transplant in the iliac fossa offers easier access through the anterior abdominal wall for tract dilation. The collecting system can be localized easily with ultrasound guidance, especially when hydronephrosis is present. This route may also handle the urologic complications of transplantation [25].

Anatomic Variations

SWL should be the first-line therapy for stones in pelvic or dystopic kidneys [26]. In cases of failure, laparoscopic assistance is essential for performing stone removal without injury to surrounding organs [12, 27, 28]. After the pneumoperitoneum is located and the external ureteral catheter is in the renal pelvis, the bowel should be displaced superiorly. Care should be taken to avoid aberrant vessels that surround the pelvis of the ectopic kidney. A pyelotomy can be performed with scissors or a knife, and the stones removed from the renal pelvis with a combination of instruments: graspers, stone baskets, and a suction probe. The ureteral catheter is then flushed with saline to clear any residual fragments. A flexible cystoscope or ureteroscope is a useful tool to locate hidden stones. Ideally, the pyelotomy is closed with sutures. However, if this is not possible owing to location, an internal double-J catheter should be inserted along with a bladder catheter for 2 weeks to promote closure of the pyelotomy. A suction drain is positioned in the perinephric area through a working port to prevent urine leak. The abdomen is exited in the standard fashion.

Calculi in pelvic kidneys involving more than the renal pelvis can be removed by PNL under laparoscopic guidance [29–31]. Once the kidney is exposed, the nephrostomy tract is created either retrograde [32] or antegrade. The ureter of a pelvic kidney is tortuous, and retrograde access to the calyx may be difficult. For the antegrade approach, puncture of the stone-bearing calyx is fluoroscopically guided, and the tract is dilated with either sequential dilators (metal or flexible) or an Amplatz balloon dilator, which may be easier. PNL is performed using standard techniques [33]. A nephrostomy tube can be left in place and brought out through a port site. Alternatively, the nephrostomy site can be sutured closed and a ureteral stent left in place.

PNL for calculi in horseshoe kidneys has been performed with success [34]. In fact, ESWL may be more difficult for two reasons. First, the anteromedial and inferior position of the horseshoe kidney makes it more difficult to focus the shockwave therapy. Second, stones in the medial calices may be obscured by the spine, and the pelvic bones may obscure the lower caliceal stones. Modifications must be made to the PNL technique because of these anatomical problems [35]. The lower abdominal position of a horseshoe kidney necessitates upper or middle caliceal puncture, while malrotation requires a more posterior puncture. Monitoring of the tract formation is difficult using fluoroscopy. Ultrasound guidance may be more helpful in this regard, and is also useful in locating aberrant vessels. The renal pelvis is deep, and a long nephroscope may be required.

Pediatric Nephrolithiasis

It is reasonable to treat children with renal lithiasis and associated anatomical abnormalities with open surgery and correction of the obstruction. However, in children who are prone to recurrence, a minimally invasive approach should be considered. SWL has been used successfully in children with a small stone burden, but general anesthesia is required and there is the potential for renal or pulmonary damage. Several reports demonstrate the safety and efficacy of PNL in children [36, 37]. The tracts were dilated to 24–26 Fr and standard nephroscopes were used. Jackman et al. [38] have described a "mini-perc" technique using an 11 Fr peel-away vascular access sheath with a 7 Fr rigid pediatric cystoscope and a 9.5 Fr flexible ureteroscope. Stone fragmentation was accomplished with a electrohydraulic probe, and stone fragments were removed via irrigation or grasping forceps. A nephroureteral stent was left indwelling, and if the nephrostogram on postoperative day 2 showed no extravasation or residual stone, the stent was removed. This technique was successful in 85% of patients, and no patient required transfusion, developed urosepsis, or had a procedure-related complication.

Urolithiasis During Pregnancy

Stones during pregnancy are a rare occurrence. If they occur, they represent a diagnostic as well as a therapeutic challenge. There are many conditions during pregnancy that mimic the symptoms of urolithiasis. Most patients will present with unresolving urinary tract infection, flank pain, and/or hematuria. Ultrasonography is the primary means of diagnosis. Transvaginal ultrasound is also helpful to image the distal ureters. When the ultrasound is equivocal, a limited intravenous pyelogram provides additional information with minimal risk to the developing fetus. The risk of radiation exposure during this examination is certainly less than the potential problems that can occur if the correct diagnosis is missed. Once the stone has been localized, the majority of pregnant patients will pass the calculus spontaneously with conservative measures alone. In those patients with unresolving pain, renal failure, or sepsis, an algorithm can be followed to manage the stone [39]. Shockwave lithotripsy is absolutely contraindicated during pregnancy. Ureteroscopic manipulation is also not indicated because of the risks of preterm delivery of the infant. Our first choice is placement of an internal ureteral stent under limited fluoroscopic or ultrasound guidance. This can be performed under sedation or regional anesthesia. The stent should be changed approximately every 4 weeks to prevent severe encrustation, as is seen during pregnancy. If the risk of stent exchange is high, consideration can be given to leaving it in for the remainder of gestation if the patient is in the third trimester. If the stent cannot be placed, a percutaneous nephrostomy is the next step. This, however, is our last resort because of the discomfort it gives the patient and the potential for urinary tract infection when left in long-term. Once the obstruction is treated, the stone can be treated postpartum using any standard technique.

Calculi in Solitary Kidneys or Bilateral Calculi

Patients with solitary kidneys are able to have PNL without any increased risk [40]. Renal function is not adversely affected, and PNL may be performed even with renal insufficiency. Care must be taken to monitor the irrigation fluid balance at all times, as these patients may not be able to handle the fluid shifts.

Once proficiency is achieved for unilateral PNL, simultaneous bilateral PNL can be performed safely [41, 42]. We tell all patients that the second-side procedure will be postponed if there are problems with the first side. Morbidity is similar to the unilateral procedure, with hospital days about the same.

Urolithiasis with Morbid Obesity

Morbid obesity may preclude the use of SWL because of weight restrictions or inability to target the stone. There are several techniques that can assist in performing PNL safely in these difficult patients. After dilating the nephrostomy tract and allowing it to mature, flexible instruments can be used for most stones. If a rigid instrument is needed for larger stones, the flank incision can be extended and the nephroscope pushed a few centimeters into the flank. Giblin et al. [43] used a longer Amplatz access sheath and a 30 Fr gynecologic laparoscope, in conjunction with extralong bronchoscopic grasping forceps, to remove stone fragments. The prone position may cause ventilatory difficulties, necessitating a flank position for PNL [44]. When using balloon dilators in morbidly obese patients, sequential dilation may be required to ensure complete tract dilation. Despite the technical difficulties, PNL in obese patients can be performed with stone-free rates and morbidity comparable to those of an unselected population [45].

Conclusion

In the United States, the treatment of stone disease may be more invasive than in other countries, possibly because of the ready availability of equipment. This is a reasonable approach if it can be done with minimal morbidity. However, it is possible that in the future, economic and time factors, as well as patient expectations, could play a stronger role worldwide in the decision-making process. Ultimately, most urinary stones can be treated with minimally invasive techniques.

References

1. Segura JW, Patterson DE, LeRoy AJ, Williams HJ, Barrett DM, Benson RJ, May GR, Bender CE (1985) Percutaneous removal of kidney stones: review of 1000 cases. J Urol 134:1077–1081
2. Lam HS, Lingeman JE, Barron M, Newman DM, Mosbaugh PG, Steele RE, Knapp PM, Scott JW, Nyhuis A, Woods JR (1992) Staghorn calculi: analysis of treatment results between initial percutaneous nephrostolithotomy and extracorporeal shockwave lithotripsy monotherapy with reference to surface area. J Urol 147:1219–1225
3. Lingeman JE, Siegel YI, Steele B, Nyhuis AW, Woods JR (1994) Management of lower pole nephrolithiasis: a critical analysis. J Urol 151:663–667
4. Cass AS (1996) Extracorporeal shockwave lithotripsy or percutaneous nephrolithotomy for lower pole nephrolithiasis? J Endourol 10:17–20
5. Elbahnasy AM, Clayman R, Shalhav L, Hoenig DM, Chandhoke PS, Lingeman JE, Denstedt JD, Kahn RI, Assimos DG, Nakada SY (1998) Lower-pole caliceal stone clearance after shockwave lithotripsy, percutaneous nephrolithotomy, and flexible ureteroscopy: impact of radiographic spatial anatomy. J Endourol 12:113–119
6. Keeley FX, Moussa SA, Smith G, Tolley DA (1999) Clearance of lower pole stones following shockwave lithotripsy: effect of the infundibulopelvic angle. Eur Urol 36:371–375
7. Segura JW (1997) Staghorn calculi. [Review] Urol Clin North Am 24:71–80
8. Segura JW, Preminger GM, Assimos DG, Dretler SP, Kahn RI, Lingeman JE, Macaluso JJ, McCullough DL (1994) Nephrolithiasis Clinical Guidelines Panel summary report on the management of staghorn calculi. American Urological Association Nephrolithiasis Clinical Guidelines Panel. J Urol 151:1648–1651
9. Streem SB (1997) Sandwich therapy. [Review]. Urol Clin North Am 24:213–223
10. Meretyk S, Gofrit ON, Gafni O, Pode D, Shapiro A, Verstandig A, Sasson T, Katz G, Landau EH (1997) Complete staghorn calculi: random prospective comparison between extracorporeal shockwave lithotripsy monotherapy and combined with percutaneous nephrostolithotomy. J Urol 157:780–786
11. Ruckle HC, Segura JW (1994) Laparoscopic treatment of a stone-filled, caliceal diverticulum: a definitive, minimally invasive therapeutic option. J Urol 151:122–124
12. Harmon WJ, Kleer E, Segura JW (1996) Laparoscopic pyelolithotomy for calculus removal in a pelvic kidney. J Urol 155:2019–2020
13. Van CJ, Abi AS, Lorge F, Wese FX, Opsomer R (1995) Laparoscopic nephrolithotomy: the value of intracorporeal sonography and color Doppler. Urology 45:516–519
14. Hoznek A, Herard A, Ogiez N, Amsellem D, Chopin DK, Abbou CC (1998) Symptomatic caliceal diverticula treated with extraperitoneal laparoscopic marsupialization fulguration and gelatin resorcinol formaldehyde glue obliteration. J Urol 160:352–355
15. Anderson KR, Keetch DW, Albala DM, Chandhoke PS, McClennan BL, Clayman RV (1994) Optimal therapy of the distal ureteral stone: extracorporeal shockwave lithotripsy versus ureteroscopy. J Urol 152:62–65
16. Pearle MS, Blackstone S, Dunn MD, Figenshau RS, Sundaram CP, McDougall EM, Clayman R, Nadler RB (1999) Prospective, randomized trial comparing ureteroscopy and shockwave lithotripsy for distal ureteral calculi. J Endourol 13(Suppl 1):42
17. Biri H, Kupeli B, Isen K, Sinik Z, Karaoglan U, Bozkirli I (1999) Treatment of lower ureteral stones: extracorporeal shockwave lithotripsy or intracorporeal lithotripsy? J Endourol 13:77–81

18. Grasso M, Loisides P, Beaghler M, Bagley D (1995) The case for primary endoscopic management of upper urinary tract calculi. 1. A critical review of 121 extracorporeal shockwave lithotripsy failures. Urology 45:363–371
19. Grasso M, Beaghler M, Loisides P (1995) The case for primary endoscopic management of upper urinary tract calculi. 2. Cost and outcome assessment of 112 primary ureteral calculi. Urology 45:372–376
20. Kapoor DA, Leech JE, Yap WT, Rose JF, Kabler R, Mowad JJ (1992) Cost and efficacy of extracorporeal shockwave lithotripsy versus ureteroscopy in the treatment of lower ureteral calculi. J Urol 148:1095–1096
21. Wolf JS, Carroll PR, Stoller ML (1995) Cost-effectiveness v patient preference in the choice of treatment for distal ureteral calculi: a literature-based decision analysis. J Endourol 9:243–248
22. Fahlenkamp D, Oesterwitz H, Althaus P, Schopke WD, Brien G (1988) Percutaneous management of urolithiasis after kidney transplantation. Report of a case and review of the literature. [Review] Eur Urol 14:330–332
23. Bailey IS, Griffin P, Evans C, Matthews PN (1989) Percutaneous surgery of the transplanted kidney. Br J Urol 63:327–328
24. Minon CJ, Garcia TE, Garcia DE, Vela NR, Ald DA, Plaza J, Alferez C (1991) Percutaneous nephrolithotomy in transplanted kidney. Urology 38:232–234
25. Gedroyc WM, MacIver D, Joyce MR, Saxton HM (1989) Percutaneous stone and stent removal from renal transplants. Clin Radiol 40:174–177
26. Lingeman JE, Smith LH, Woods JR, Newman DM (1987) Extracorporeal shockwave lithotripsy. In: Urinary calculi: ESWL, endourology, and medical therapy. Lea and Febiger, Philadelphia, p 366
27. Chang TD, Dretler SP (1996) Laparoscopic pyelolithotomy in an ectopic kidney. J Urol 156:1753
28. Figge M (1988) Percutaneous transperitoneal nephrolithotomy. Eur Urol 14:414–416
29. Zafar FS, Lingeman JE (1996) Value of laparoscopy in the management of calculi complicating renal malformations. J Endourol 10:379–383
30. Holman E, Toth C (1998) Laparoscopically assisted percutaneous transperitoneal nephrolithotomy in pelvic dystopic kidneys: experience in 15 successful cases. J Laparoendosc Adv Surg Tech A 8:431–435
31. Toth C, Holman E, Pasztor I, Khan AM (1993) Laparoscopically controlled and assisted percutaneous transperitoneal nephrolithotomy in a pelvic dystopic kidney. J Endourol 7:303–305
32. Eshghi AM, Roth JS, Smith AD (1985) Percutaneous transperitoneal approach to a pelvic kidney for endourological removal of staghorn calculus. J Urol 134:525–527
33. Segura JW, LeRoy AJ (1984) Percutaneous ultrasonic lithotripsy. Urology 23:7–10
34. Jones DJ, Wickham JE, Kellett MJ (1991) Percutaneous nephrolithotomy for calculi in horseshoe kidneys. J Urol 145:481–483
35. Cussenot O, Desgrandchamps F, Ollier P, Teillac P, Le DA (1992) Anatomical bases of percutaneous surgery for calculi in horseshoe kidney. Surg Radiol Anat 14:209–213
36. Mor Y, Elmasry YE, Kellet MJ, Duffy PG (1997) The role of percutaneous nephrolithotomy in the management of pediatric renal calculi. J Urol 158:1319–1321
37. Kurzrock EA, Huffman JL, Hardy BE, Fugelso P (1996) Endoscopic treatment of pediatric urolithiasis. J Pediatr Surg 31:1413–1416
38. Jackman SV, Hedican SP, Peters CA, Docimo SG (1998) Percutaneous nephrolithotomy in infants and preschool age children: experience with a new technique. Urology 52:697–701

39. Hendricks SK, Ross SO, Krieger JN (1991) An algorithm for diagnosis and therapy of management and complications of urolithiasis during pregnancy. Surg Gynecol Obstet 172:49–54
40. Jones DJ, Kellett MJ, Wickham JE (1991) Percutaneous nephrolithotomy and the solitary kidney. J Urol 145:477–479
41. Dushinski JW, Lingeman JE (1997) Simultaneous bilateral percutaneous nephrolithotomy. J Urol 158:2065–2068
42. Ahlawat R, Banerjee GK, Dalela D (1995) Bilateral simultaneous percutaneous nephrolithotomy. A prospective feasibility study. Eur Urol 28:116–118
43. Giblin JG, Lossef S, Pahira JJ (1995) A modification of the standard percutaneous nephrolithotripsy technique for the morbidly obese patient. Urology 46:491–493
44. Faerber GJ, Goh M (1997) Percutaneous nephrolithotripsy in the morbidly obese patient. Tech Urol 3:89–95
45. Pearle MS, Nakada SY, Womack JS, Kryger JV (1998) Outcomes of contemporary percutaneous nephrostolithotomy in morbidly obese patients. J Urol 160:669–673

Epidemiology of Urolithiasis in Japan

Akito Terai and Osamu Yoshida

Summary. Retrospective nationwide surveys of urolithiasis in Japan were conducted in 1955, 1966, 1979, 1990, and 1999, and covered nearly all the urologists practicing in Japan. In the years of interest, all outpatient visits to urologists which resulted in a diagnosis of urinary tract stones were enumerated, irrespective of admission or treatment. A comprehensive review of these surveys has shed light on the changing pattern of urolithiasis in Japan during the 20th century.

Upper urinary tract stones, which accounted for 40%–60% of cases until 1945, have steadily increased to 97% in 1995. Male preponderance decreased from 7:1 in 1935 to 2.5:1 in 1965 and thereafter. The annual incidence (per 100000) of upper urinary tract stones has steadily increased from 43.7 in 1965 to 80.9 in 1995. This steady increase over the past 30 years will continue in the near future, but it is still lower than that in the United States. The life-long risk of upper urinary tract stones in 1995 was estimated to be 9.0% for men and 3.8% for women. Lower urinary tract stones are predominant in men ≥ 60 years of age. The annual incidence of lower urinary tract stones has decreased from 37.2 to 27.0 in men (≥ 60 years old) and increased from 2.4 to 4.8 in women (≥ 60 years old). Stone composition recorded by infrared spectroscopy showed that an increase in calcium oxalate and uric acid stones and a decrease in calcium phosphate and infection stones is a phenomenon which is common to both upper and lower urinary tract stones.

Key Words. Urinary calculi, Nationwide survey, Epidemiology, Annual incidence, Stone composition

Department of Urology, Faculty of Medicine, Kyoto University, Sakyo-ku, Kyoto 606-8507, Japan

Introduction

Urolithiasis is known to have occurred for thousands of years BC. Until the 19th century, urolithiasis in Europe seems to have been almost exclusively bladder stones. In industrialized countries in North America and Europe, as well as in Japan, the incidence of bladder stones has strongly decreased during the 20th century, while calcium-containing kidney stones have markedly increased. Bladder stones only account for about 10% of all urinary stones in industrialized countries, but they remain an important cause of morbidity in certain parts of middle and southeast Asia [1].

In Japan, nationwide hospital surveys of urolithiasis were conducted in 1955 [2], 1966 [3], 1979 [4], 1990 [5], and 1999 [6], and have clearly demonstrated the changing pattern of urolithiasis in the Japanese population in the last half of the 20th century. The incidence of urolithiasis in Japan has steadily increased since World War II, as it has in other developed countries in Europe and in the United States [7]. During the full industrialization of Japan over the last few decades, life style and dietary habits have been dramatically Westernized. Idiopathic calcium urolithiasis in the upper urinary tract has become by far the most common type of urinary calculi. Extracorporeal shock-wave lithotripsy and endourological treatments such as percutaneous nephrolithotripsy and transurethral reterolithotripsy, begun in Japan in 1984, fundamentally changed stone treatments in subsequent years [6]. Furthermore, Japan is the world's most rapidly aging society, and this aging is a comparatively recent phenomenon, first observed in the 1970s.

This chapter provides a comprehensive review of the nationwide surveys of urolithiasis in Japan, and considers the changing pattern in the 20th century. For detailed epidemiological aspects of urolithiasis, such as age, sex, family history, geography, climatic and seasonal factors, diet, and water intake, readers should refer to other excellent reviews and papers [8–11].

Survey Methods

With the cooperation of the Japanese Urological Association, all major hospitals were invited to participate in nationwide surveys of urolithiasis. The surveys of 1955, 1966, 1979, and 1990 included all general hospitals with ≥200 inpatient beds and a urological department, while the survey of 1999 enrolled all hospitals approved by the Japanese Board of Urology (i.e., general hospitals with ≥100 inpatient beds, including ≥15 beds in a urological department, or urological clinics with ≥50 inpatient beds). These criteria covered nearly all practicing urologists in Japan.

In this retrospective survey, the enrolled hospitals were asked by postal questionnaire to investigate all outpatient visits that resulted in a diagnosis of urolithiasis in each survey year. The diagnostic criterion of urolithiasis was defined as radiographic and/or endoscopic confirmation of calculi. Patients with only a history of stone passage were excluded from the study. Urologists practicing in the enrolled hospitals reviewed the medical charts and abstracted the data. The survey questionnaire included items on the age and sex of the stone patients, the locations of the stones (upper or lower urinary tract, or both), and whether the stones had developed for the first time in the patient's life. All the stone patients were enumerated, whether or not they were hospitalized or had treatment, and the number of patients seen in each institution was entered in the survey questionnaire according to the items investigated.

The total number of patients in Japan was estimated by the formula

$$\text{Number of patients reported} \times \frac{\text{Total number of beds in the enrolled hospitals}}{\text{Total number of beds in the respondent hospitals}}$$

Our estimation did not include stone patients seen only in private physicians' offices, but we presumed that the majority of patients with urolithiasis in Japan were diagnosed and treated by urologists. The annual incidence was calculated as the estimated number of stone patients per 100000 of the general population. Data from the Population Census of Japan were used for this purpose. In the estimations of annual incidence, upper urinary tract stones included only first-episode stones, while lower urinary tract stones included both first-episode and recurrent stones. Life-long risk of urolithiasis was estimated by multiplying the annual incidence by the life expectancy at birth in any given year.

Location of Calculi

Upper urinary tract stones accounted for 40%–60% of cases before 1945. After World War II, the frequency of upper urinary tract stones steadily increased to 95% in 1965 and, most recently, as high as 97% in 1995 (Fig. 1).

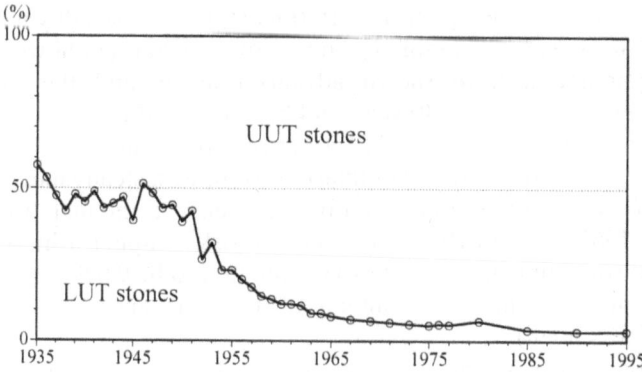

FIG. 1. Chronological changes in the ratio of upper (*UUT*) to lower (*LUT*) urinary tract stones in Japan from 1935 to 1995

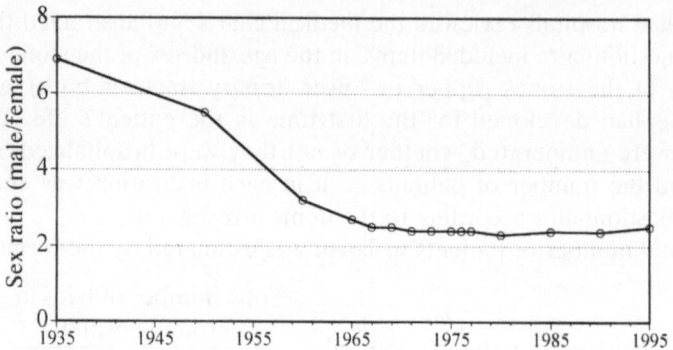

FIG. 2. Chronological changes in the sex ratio of urolithiasis in Japan from 1935 to 1995, including both upper and lower urinary tract stones

Sex and Age Distribution

The male preponderance of urolithiasis decreased from 7:1 in 1935 to 2.5:1 in 1965, and has remained steady since 1965 (Fig. 2).

The age distribution for upper urinary tract stones showed that the peak age has shifted from the twenties and thirties in men and the twenties in women in 1965, to the forties in men and the fifties in women in 1995 (Fig. 3a). Lower urinary tract stones are predominant in elderly people in both sexes. The small peaks shown in the twenties and thirties in 1965 have disappeared by 1995 (Fig. 3b).

Annual Incidence of Upper Urinary Tract Stones

Annual incidences (per 100000 population) have been calculated for both upper and lower urinary tract stones in the years 1965, 1975, 1985, and 1995. The annual incidence of first-episode upper urinary tract stones has steadily increased from 43.7 in 1965 to 80.9 in 1995 (Table 1). During the last 30 years, however, the entire Japanese population have shown advanced aging, and the proportion of Japanese men and women ≥ 40 years old has increased from 27.8% and 31.5%, respectively, in 1965 to 48.0% and 51.9%, respectively, in 1995 (Fig. 4). The age-adjusted annual incidence of urothithiasis also shows a steady increase from 54.2 in 1965 to 68.9 in 1995, accompanied by a decrease in the male to female ratio from 2.8 in 1965 to 1.8 in 1995 (Table 1). The risk of upper urinary tract stones occurring at some time in one's life was estimated to be 9.0% for men and 3.8% for women in 1995, which is a doubling of the value since 1965 (4.3% for men and 1.8% for women).

The chronological changes in the sex- and age-related annual incidence between 1965 and 1995 showed that in men, the peak age of first-episode upper urinary tract stones has shifted from the twenties, thirties, and forties in 1965 to

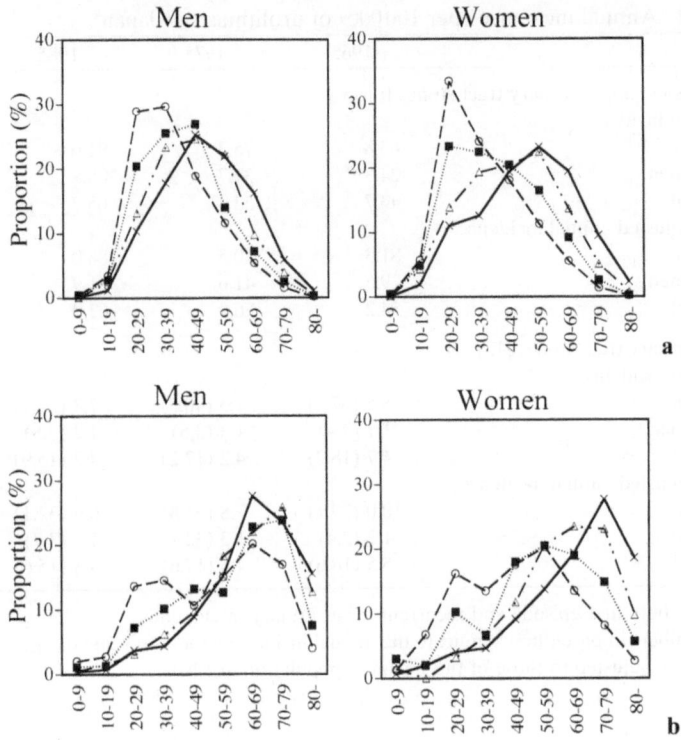

Fig. 3. Chronological changes in the age and sex distribution of urolithiasis in Japan from 1965 to 1995. **a** Upper urinary tract stones; **b** lower urinary tract stones. *Circles*, 1965; *squares*, 1975; *triangles*, 1985; *crosses*, 1995

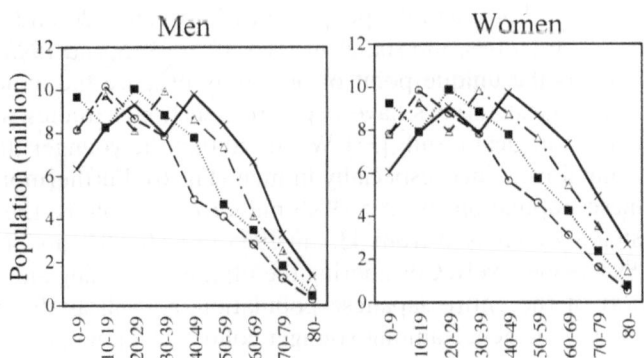

Fig. 4. Chronological changes in the age and sex distribution of the entire Japanese census population from 1965 to 1995. *Circles*, 1965; *squares*, 1975; *triangles*, 1985; *crosses*, 1995

TABLE 1. Annual incidence (per 100000) of urolithiasis in Japan[a]

	1965	1975	1985	1995
First-episode upper urinary tract stones [6]				
Annual incidence				
Men	63.8	75.7	91.6	117.5
Women	24.3	31.7	40.8	46.1
Total	43.7	53.4	65.7	80.9
Age-adjusted annual incidence[c]				
Men	81.3	80.5	86.0	100.1
Women	29.5	41.6	51.9	55.4
Total	54.2	56.4	62.0	68.9
Lower urinary tract stones [12][b]				
Annual incidence				
Men	8.5 (37.2)	7.3 (40.3)	7.3 (32.7)	9.8 (27.0)
Women	1.1 (2.4)	1.3 (3.5)	1.2 (3.8)	2.2 (4.8)
Total	4.7 (18.2)	4.2 (17.2)	4.2 (15.9)	5.9 (14.4)
Age-adjusted annual incidence[c]				
Men	10.0 (39.1)	7.8 (35.8)	6.6 (32.1)	7.0 (34.6)
Women	1.2 (2.4)	1.3 (3.5)	1.1 (3.7)	1.6 (5.9)
Total	5.5 (18.6)	4.5 (17.6)	3.8 (15.6)	4.3 (18.1)

[a] Includes both first-episode and recurrent lower urinary tract stones.
[b] The numbers in parentheses indicate the annual incidences for ≥60 years of age.
[c] Ages were adjusted to those of the Japanese population in 1980.

the thirties, forties, and fifties in 1995 (Fig. 5a). In women, the peak age of the twenties in 1965 had shifted to the fifties and sixties by 1995. Whereas the annual incidence has remained relatively constant over the past 30 years for people in their first decade, teens, and twenties, there is a continuous increase after the age of 30.

Because the past and present nationwide surveys of urolithiasis investigated the annual incidence for the entire Japanese population, we could calculate 30-year longitudinal changes in the annual incidence for defined cohorts in that population (Fig. 6). For example, people born between 1926 and 1935 were in their thirties, forties, fifties, and sixties in 1965, 1975, 1985, and 1995, respectively (group ④). This is the unique point of our study because the majority of published epidemiological surveys have been cross-sectional studies which did not account for chronological trends [13]. We found that the younger the cohort, the higher the annual incidence, especially in men (Fig. 6). Furthermore, taking the entire Japanese population in 1965 (98.3 million) as a cohort, the annual incidence has steadily increased from 43.7 in 1965 to 64.0, 88.9, and 110.9 in 1975, 1985, and 1995, respectively. Considering the rapidly increasing annual incidence for the cohort of the entire Japanese population, as well as the progressively increasing annual incidence among younger cohort groupings, there is sufficient evidence to predict that the occurrence of upper urinary tract stones will continue to increase in the near future. Furthermore, the peak age for first-episode upper urinary tract stones has moved toward older people (Fig. 6). Elderly

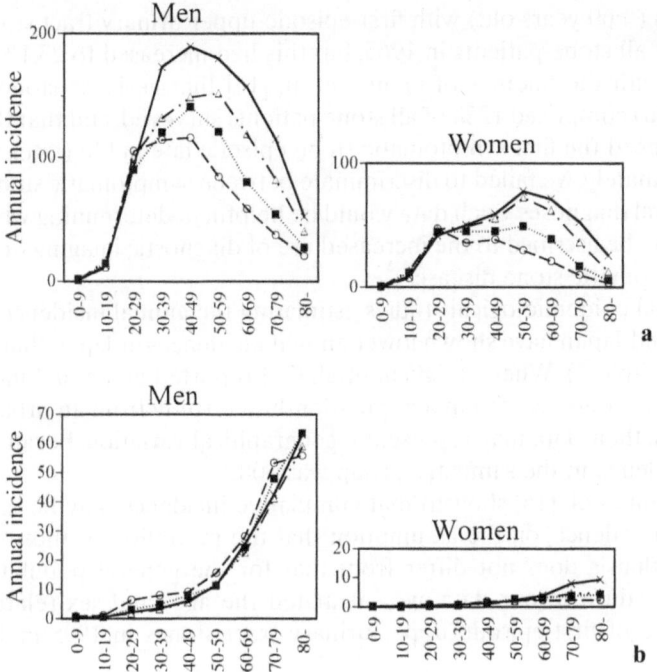

Fig. 5. Chronological changes in age- and sex-related annual incidence of urolithiasis (per 100000) in Japan from 1965 to 1995. **a** Upper urinary tract stones (only first-episode stones); **b** lower urinary tract stones (both first-episode and recurrent stones). *Circles,* 1965; *squares,* 1975; *triangles,* 1985; *crosses,* 1995

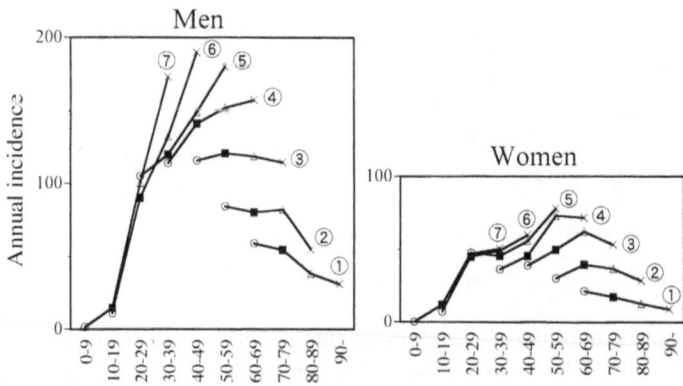

Fig. 6. Longitudinal changes in the annual incidence of upper urinary tract stones (per 100000) among different generations. *Circles,* 1965; *squares,* 1975; *triangles,* 1985; *crosses,* 1995. The numbers in circles indicate generations born in different periods: *1,* 1896–1905; *2,* 1906–1915; *3,* 1916–1925; *4,* 1926–1935; *5,* 1936–1945; *6,* 1946–1955; *7,* 1956–1965

patients (≥60 years old) with first-episode upper urinary tract stones comprised 7.1% of all stone patients in 1965, but this had increased to 23.1% by 1995. This agrees with the findings of Gentle et al. [14] that geriatric stone formers (>65 years old) comprised 12% of all stone patients surveyed, and that they commonly experienced the first symptomatic stone episode late in life (after the age of 50). Unfortunately, we failed to discriminate between symptomatic stone patients and incidental diagnoses. Such data would be helpful in determining whether the time trend can be ascribed to the increased use of diagnostic imaging or to an increase in symptomatic stone disease.

Several epidemiological studies estimating the annual incidence in the United States and Japan have shown lower annual incidences in Japan than in the United States (Table 2). Whereas Iguchi et al. [22] reported an annual incidence of 971 per 100000 (ages 20–59) in a population-based study from an urban satellite city in Japan, their data may represent a geographical variation, because in our study the incidence in the same age group was 108.

Johnson et al. [16] showed that cumulative incidence may be used to approximate prevalence, on the assumption that the mortality for those with a history of urolithiasis does not differ from that for the general population. Applying this procedure to our data, we calculated the age- and sex-related cumulative incidence of first-episode upper urinary tract stones in 1995 in Japan (Fig. 7).

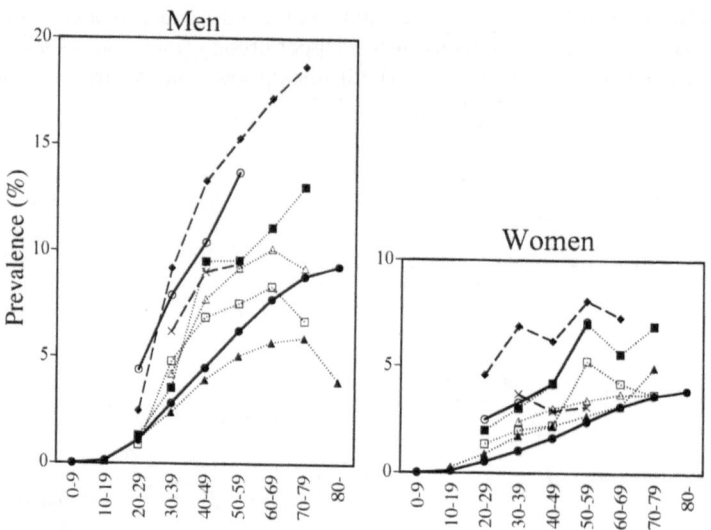

FIG. 7. Comparison of the age- and sex-related prevalence of urolithiasis (%) in population-based studies. *Closed circles*, the cumulative incidence calculated from the 1995 data in Japan [6]. *Open circles*, prevalences in Kaizuka, Japan in 1992 [22]; *closed triangles*, prevalences in Northern California, USA, between 1970 and 1972 [17]. Prevalences throughout the USA are shown by *open squares* (between 1976 and 1980 [24]), *open triangles* (in 1982 [25]), and *closed squares* (between 1988 and 1994 [24]). *Closed diamonds*, prevalences in Denmark in 1959 [26]; *crosses*, prevalences in Stockholm, Sweden, in 1977 [27]

TABLE 2. Estimates of the annual incidence of urinary calculi in the United States and Japan

Reference	Year(s) studied	Country	Area	Method	Sex[a]	Age	Stone location[b]	Annual incidence[c]
Boyce et al. [15]	1952	USA	Nationwide	Hospital survey	B	All	B	94.7
Johnson et al. [16]	1950–1974	USA	Rochester, MN	Medical records	B	≥10	U	58.7–73.4
					M	≥10	U	78.5–123.6
					F	≥10	U	32.4–43.2
Hiatt et al. [17]	1970–1972	USA	Northern California	Medical records	B	All	B	122
					M	All	B	181
					F	All	B	59
Sierakowski et al. [18]	1974	USA	Nationwide	Hospital survey	B	All	B	164
Schey et al. [19]	1977	USA	Forsyth County, NC	Medical records	B	All	U	208
Thun and Schober [20]	1991	USA	Tennessee	Cohort study	M	30–69	U	421
Curhan et al. [21]	1986–1992	USA	Nationwide	Cohort study	M	40–75	U	273–326
Iguchi et al. [22]	1992	Japan	Kaizuka City (urban)	Population-based study	B	20–59	B	971
Takeuchi et al. [23]	1991–1993	Japan	Tajima area (rural)	Medical records	B	All	B	93
Yoshida et al. [6]	1995	Japan	Nationwide	Hospital survey	B	All	U	80.9[d]
					M	All	U	115.8[d]
					F	All	U	46.9[d]

[a] M, male; F, female; B, both sexes.
[b] U, upper urinary tract stones; B, both upper and lower urinary tract calculi.
[c] Annual incidence per 100000.
[d] Not age-adjusted.

Figure 7 also shows the age- and sex-related prevalence of urolithiasis reported in various population-based surveys. The estimated prevalences among the age groups defined show a gradual increase from 3.6% and 1.4% in 1965 among men and women (ages ≥ 30), respectively, to 5.2% and 2.1% in 1995, although these figures are undoubtedly underestimated.

Annual Incidence of Lower Urinary Tract Stones

Both first-episode and recurrent stones were included in the estimation of the annual incidence of lower urinary tract stones. The chronological changes in the sex- and age-related annual incidence of lower urinary tract stones are shown in Fig. 5b. It is evident that lower urinary tract stones are predominant in men ≥ 60 years of age, and that the annual incidence increases progressively with age in both sexes. Whereas the age distribution of the annual incidence in men has been remarkably constant for the past 30 years, a progressive increase was observed in women ≥ 60 years of age. Between 1965 and 1995, the annual incidence of lower urinary tract stones for people ≥ 60 years of age decreased from 37.2 to 27.0 in men and increased from 2.4 to 4.8 in women (Table 1). The male to female ratio decreased from 7.7 to 4.5 during this interval. The male and female population ≥ 60 years of age increased from 4.3 million (9.0% of the total male population) and 5.2 million (10.4% of the total female population), respectively, in 1965 to 11.3 million (18.4%) and 14.9 million (23.2%), respectively, in 1995 (Fig. 4).

Because it is known that the majority of bladder stones develop on the basis of predisposing factors [28, 29], one possible reason for a decreasing incidence of male lower urinary tract stones may be that a greater proportion of men with predisposing factors to vesical calculosis is seeking medical advice than ever before. According to the Patient Survey in Japan (the Statistics and Information Department, Minister's Secretariat, Ministry of Health and Welfare of Japan), the rate of patients (per 100000) ≥ 65 years of age have increased more between 1965 and 1993 (from 7813 to 17518) than that for all ages combined (from 5910 to 6735).

Composition of Upper Urinary Tract Stones

Stone composition was determined by infrared spectroscopy. Table 3 shows the chronological changes in the composition of upper urinary tract stones over the past 30 years. Calcium-containing stones (consisting of calcium oxalate and/or apatite) in women have increased from 71.3% to 82.5%, which is close to the figure in men (86.1%), although pure calcium oxalate stones have been more common in men than in women. Furthermore, a decrease in infection stones (containing struvite and/or carbonate apatite) and an increase in uric acid ($\pm$ calcium oxalate) stones have occurred in both men and women. These chronological changes are statistically significant (Table 3).

TABLE 3. Stone composition according to sex[a]

Composition	Men			Women		
	1965–1977[c]	1978–1987[c]	1995	1965–1977[c]	1978–1987[c]	1995
Upper urinary tract stones [4, 5, unpublished data]						
Calcium oxalate and/or apatite	83.7%[f]	84.5%[c]	86.1%[e,f]	71.3%[d,f]	75.0%[d,e]	82.5%[e,f]
Calcium oxalate	35.1	37.9	47.4	17.9	23.4	31.7
Apatite	4.2	2.9	1.5	9.1	7.7	5.4
Calcium oxalate and apatite	44.4	43.7	37.2	44.3	43.9	45.4
Infection stones[b]	7.5[d,f]	5.2[d,e]	2.7[e,f]	23.3[d,f]	18.3[d,e]	10.5[e,f]
Uric acid	4.6[d,f]	5.7[f]	5.6[f]	1.4[f]	1.4[e]	2.7[e,f]
Cystine	1.6	1.0	1.4	1.1	1.1	1.9
Calcium oxalate and uric acid	NA	1.5	3.3	NA	0.5	1.2
Others	2.6	2.1	0.9	2.9	3.7	1.2
	(n = 9041)	(n = 46441)	(n = 2344)	(n = 4085)	(n = 17441)	(n = 775)
Lower urinary tract stones [4, 5, 12]						
Calcium oxalate and/or apatite	50.7[d]	55.0[d]	58.8	42.7	41.7	42.9
Calcium oxalate	10.4	14.3	15.5	8.0	9.0	–
Apatite	9.6	7.9	6.5	11.7	9.2	22.9
Calcium oxalate and apatite	30.7	32.8	36.8	23.0	23.5	20.0
Infection stones[b]	26.2[d,f]	20.4[f]	14.2[f]	39.8	44.8	54.3
Uric acid	11.3[d,f]	13.9[d,e]	20.0[e,f]	2.1	2.9	–
Cystine	1.4	0.7	0.7	1.7	0.7	–
Calcium oxalate and uric acid	NA	2.1	3.9	NA	0.5	–
Others	10.4	7.9	2.3	13.7	9.4	2.8
	(n = 1243)	(n = 5119)	(n = 155)	(n = 239)	(n = 948)	(n = 35)

[a] Numbers indicate the percentage in each stone. NA, not available; –, none.
[b] Infection stones were defined as stones containing struvite and/or carbonate apatite.
[c] Data during the 1965–1977 and 1978–1987 periods were cited from references 6 and 7, respectively.
Results of a χ^2 test are as follows:
1965–1977 vs. 1978–1987: [d], statistically significant ($P < 0.02$ to $P < 0.0001$).
1978–1987 vs. 1995: [e], statistically significant ($P < 0.05$ to $P < 0.0001$).
1965–1977 vs. 1995: [f], statistically significant ($P < 0.05$ to $P < 0.0001$).

Calcium oxalate and uric acid stones have increased steadily during the past 30 years, while apatite and struvite/carbonate apatite stones have gradually decreased. This chronological trend in Japan was in agreement with comparable studies conducted in Germany, showing that calcium oxalate stones have increased from 64.5% (1970s) to 72%–73% (1990s), and struvite stones have decreased from 7.0% to 3.3%–4.2% [7]. In Germany, uric acid stones have decreased from 15.3% to 8.3%–9.5%, whereas in Japan and the United States, an increase has been observed [30, 31]. In Canada, there was a relative increase in oxalate stones (from 57% to 69%) and decrease in phosphate stones (from 18% to 14%) from the first (1980 to 1983) to the last (1995 to 1998) 4-year period studied [32]. The same tendency was also observed in Japan (Table 3).

Composition of Lower Urinary Tract Stones

The chronological changes in composition of lower urinary tract stones are shown in Table 3. In men, calcium-containing stones and uric acid stones have significantly increased from 50.7% to 58.8% and from 11.3% to 20.0%, respectively, whilst infection stones have significantly decreased from 26.2% to 14.2%. In women, however, calcium-containing stones and infection stones are two major types of lower urinary tract calculi, and no significant chronological changes were observed.

The percentages of various stone types in our study coincide with those reported by Takasaki et al. [29]. They found that calcium-containing stones, uric acid stones, and infectious stones accounted for 40.0%, 5.7%, and 50.0%, respectively, of 300 lower urinary tract calculi. Because 59 of 120 patients with calcium-containing stones had no lower urinary tract disorders, and 30 of the 59 patients had coexistent upper urinary tract calculi, it was suggested that most of these stones had descended from the kidneys [29]. An increase in calcium-containing stones and uric acid stones, as well as a decrease in infection stones, is a phenomenon common to both upper and lower urinary tract stones [12]. Furthermore, calcium-containing stones usually developed as a single stone and tended to be smaller in size than infection stones or uric acid stones [12]. Therefore, many calcium-containing stones found in the lower urinary tract may have formed in the upper urinary tract and become trapped in the bladder [29].

References

1. Asper R (1984) Epidemiology and socioeconomic aspects of urolithiasis. Urol Res 12:1–5
2. Inada T (1955) Statistical study of urolithiasis in Japan (in Japanese). Hinyokika Kiyo 1:143–152
3. Inada T (1966) Research on urolithiasis (in Japanese). Nihon Hinyokika Gakkai Zasshi 57:917–929
4. Yoshida O (1979) Epidemiology of urolithiasis in Japan (in Japanese). Nihon Hinyokika Gakkai Zasshi 70:975–983

5. Yoshida O, Okada Y (1990) Epidemiology of urolithiasis in Japan: a chronological and geographical study. Urol Int 45:104–111
6. Yoshida O, Terai A, Ohkawa T, Okada Y (1999) National trend of the incidence of urolithiasis in Japan from 1965 to 1995. Kidney Int 56:1899–1904
7. Hesse A, Siener R (1997) Current aspects of epidemiology and nutrition in urinary stone disease. World J Urol 15:165–171
8. Trinchieri A (1996) Epidemiology of urolithiasis. Arch Ital Urol 68:203–249
9. Parivar F, Low RK, Stoller ML (1996) The influence of diet on urinary stone disease. J Urol 155:432–440
10. Curhan GC, Willett WC, Rimm EB, Stampfer MJ (1993) A prospective study of dietary calcium and other nutrients and the risk of symptomatic kidney stones. N Engl J Med 328:833–838
11. Curhan G, Willett W, Rimm E, Stampfer M (1997) Family history and risk of kidney stones. J Am Soc Nephrol 8:1568–1573
12. Terai A, Okada Y, Ohkawa T, Ogawa O, Yoshida O (2000) Changes in the incidence of lower urinary tract stones in Japan from 1965 to 1995. Int J Urol 7:542–456
13. Ljunghall S (1987) Incidence of upper urinary tract stones. Miner Electr Metab 13:220–227
14. Gentle DL, Stoller ML, Bruce JE, Leslie SW (1997) Geriatric urolithiasis. J Urol 158:2221–2224
15. Boyce WH, Garvey FK, Strawcutter HE (1956) Incidence of urinary calculi among patients in general hospitals, 1948 to 1952. JAMA 161:1437–1442
16. Johnson CM, Wilson DM, O'Fallon WM, Malek RS, Kurland LT (1979) Renal stone epidemiology: a 25-year study in Rochester, Minnesota. Kidney Int 16:624–631
17. Hiatt RA, Dales LG, Friedman GD, Hunkeler EM (1982) Frequency of urolithiasis in a prepaid medical care program. Am J Epidemiol 115:255–265
18. Sierakowski R, Finlayson B, Landes RR, Finlayson CD, Sierakowski N (1978) The frequency of urolithiasis in hospital discharge diagnosis in the United States. Invest Urol 15:438–441
19. Schey HM, Corbett WT, Resnick MI (1979) Prevalence rate of renal stone disease in Forsyth County, North Carolina, during 1977. J Urol 122:288–291
20. Thun MJ, Schober S (1991) Urolithiasis in Tennessee: an occupational window into a regional problem. Am J Pub Health 81:587–591
21. Curhan GC, Rimm EB, Willett WC, Stampfer MJ (1994) Regional variation in nephrolithiasis incidence and prevalence among United States men. J Urol 151:838–841
22. Iguchi M, Umekawa T, Katoh Y, Kohri K, Kurita T (1996) Prevalence of urolithiasis in Kaizuka City, Japan: an epidemiologic study of urinary stones. Int J Urol 3:175–179
23. Takeuchi H, Yoshida H, Isogawa Y, Taki Y (1999) Prevalence of upper urinary tract stones in Tajima, North Hyogo, Japan (in Japanese). Hinyokika Kiyo 45:165–168
24. Stamatelou KK, Jones CA, Francis ME, Nyberg LM (1998) Time trends in reported prevalence of kidney stones in the USA: 1976–1994. J Urol 159:141A
25. Soucie JM, Thun MJ, Coates RJ, McClellan W, Austin H (1994) Demographic and geographic variability of kidney stones in the United States. Kidney Int 46:893–899
26. Larsen JF, Phillip J (1962) Studies on the incidence of urolithiasis. Urol Int 13:53–64
27. Ljunghall S, Christensson T, Wengle B (1977) Prevalence and incidence of renal stone disease in a health screening programme. Scand J Urol Nephrol Suppl 41:39–54
28. Douenias R, Rich M, Badlani G, Mazor D, Smith A (1991) Predisposing factors in bladder calculi. Review of 100 cases. Urology 37:240–243

29. Takasaki E, Suzuki T, Honda M, Imai T, Maeda S, Hosoya Y (1995) Chemical compositions of 300 lower urinary tract calculi and associated disorders in the urinary tract. Urol Int 54:89–94
30. Smith LH (1989) The medical aspects of urolithiasis: an overview. J Urol 141:707–710
31. Mandel NS, Mandel GS (1989) Urinary tract stone disease in the United States veteran population. II. Geographical analysis of variations in composition. J Urol 142:1516–1521
32. Gault MH, Chafe L (2000) Relationship of frequency, age, sex, stone weight and composition in 15264 stones: comparison of results for 1980 to 1983 and 1995 to 1998. J Urol 164:302–307

Urolithiasis—Patient Evaluation and Medical Treatment

David A. Lifshitz[1], Arieh L. Shalhav[2], and James E. Lingeman[1]

Summary. The surgical management of urinary stone disease has evolved in the last three decades from traditional open surgery to minimally invasive techniques including extracorporeal shock wave lithotripsy, ureteroscopy, and percutaneous surgery. Although similar dramatic advances in the medical treatment of urolithiasis have not occurred, much progress has been made in understanding factors that are important in the genesis and prevention of urinary calculi.

This chapter aims to provide a current practical set of guidelines for the assessment and medical management of patients with urolithiasis, based on the latest available information regarding pathogenesis and medical treatment options. All urolithiasis patients should undergo a basic evaluation, which is considered to be the minimal essential diagnostic workup, in order to rule out obvious, treatable systemic causes of urinary stone disease. Stone analysis, when available, should be an indispensable part of the assessment in order to identify specific types of urinary stones and allow the application of the most appropriate medical therapy. Every patient should be advised about conservative nonspecific preventative measures. High-risk calcium stone patients should have a more extensive metabolic evaluation based on two 24-h urine samples.

Key Words. Metabolic evaluation, Urolithiasis, Idiopathic hypercalciuria, Struvite, Cystinuria

Introduction

Renal stone disease accounts for about 7–10 of every 1000 hospital admissions in the United States [1]. Between 5% and 15% of the population will develop kidney stones during their lifetime [2]. Although stones are more common

[1] Methodist Hospital Institute for Kidney Stone Disease, 1801 North Senate Blvd., Suite 220, Indianapolis, IN 46202, USA
[2] Department of Urology, Indiana University School of Medicine, USA

in men, the incidence in women appears to be increasing. In both sexes, the peak age of onset is during the third and fourth decade of life. There has been an increase in the prevalence of calcium stones in industrialized countries [3].

Kidney stones cause considerable suffering and have a substantial economic impact. In 1993, the total annual cost for urolithiasis treatment in the United States was estimated to be $1.83 billion [4]. Surgical treatment, including lithotripsy, is not a substitute for medical prevention which has been proven to be effective in reducing stone recurrence [5]. Medical prevention based on the appropriate evaluation and treatment of metabolically active stone disease could save nearly $2200 per patient per year in related re-treatment costs [6]. An understanding of the factors leading to stone formation and a structured patient evaluation are the bases for effective medical prevention. In this chapter, general principles and guidelines will be presented for the initial medical and laboratory evaluation of a patient with urinary stones.

Risk of Stone Recurrence

The risk of recurrence, as studied in a large series of first-time stone formers, has been reported to be about 67% after 9 years [7]; after 25 years, 75% of patients have formed a second stone [8]. Recurrence rates are higher in patients with recurrent stones or patients forming multiple stones, and can reach 50% in 3 years [9].

Pathogenesis of Stone Disease

Kidney stones are generally composed of calcium salts, uric acid, magnesium ammonium phosphate, or cystine (Table 1). Most calcium oxalate stones also contain a small amount of hydroxyapatite and 10%–12% contain some uric acid.

Kidney stones (especially those composed of calcium salts) result from a complex physical and chemical process. Two major opposing forces are the

TABLE 1. Frequency of various types of stone [10]

Stone type	% of total
Calcium Oxalate	58.8
Mixed CaO_x with calcium phosphate	11.4
Uric acid	10.1
Struvite	9.3
Calcium phosphate	8.9
Miscellaneous	0.8
Cystine	0.7

key factors in stone formation. On the one hand urinary supersaturation (SS) provides the driving force for stone formation, while on the other hand, urine inhibitors provide a protective effect. Stones form in urine that is supersaturated with respect to the ionic components of the specific stone. SS means that the concentration of a stone-forming salt, such as calcium oxalate, exceeds its solubility in a solution (the solubility product), and once reached, nuclei of its solid phase can form. In urine, SS may rise to between two-fold and eight-fold, depending upon the crystal involved, without new solid-phase formation. This zone is termed the "metastable zone." At SS values above the upper limit of the metastable zone (termed the formation product), crystal nuclei will form spontaneously, grow, and aggregate (Fig. 1). Urinary SS of a particular crystal component has been shown to correlate directly with the stone type that the individual develops [11]. Solute urine concentration is a function of how much of the particular ion is excreted in the volume of urine. Thus, increased urinary ion concentration and decreased urine volume will both increase free ion activity and favor stone formation and growth. In some cases, high SS is the only apparent reason for stones. Cystine, struvite, and uric acid stones are typical examples of stone formation driven by high SS and will be discussed separately.

Unstable Zone: 　　CaOx: SS>8 　　Brushite: SS>2.5 　　Uric Acid: SS>2	Nuclei form, grow, and aggregate
Metastable Upper Limit: Formation Product	**First solid phase formation**
Metastable Zone: 　　CaOx: 1<SS<8 　　Brushite: 1<SS<2.5 　　Uric Acid: 1<SS<2	**Spontaneous nucleation does not occur** **Crystal growth can occur** **Inhibitors can impede or prevent crystallization**
Equilibrium Point: Solubility Product 　　SS = 1	Crystals neither grow nor dissolve
Undersaturation Zone: 　　SS < 1	Nuclei may dissolve (uric acid)

FIG. 1. Effects of increased solute concentration

TABLE 2. Urinary inhibitors [12–21]

Inorganic Inhibitors
Pyrophosphate
Magnesium

Organic inhibitors
Citrate
Tamm–Horsfall protein
Uropontin
Nephrocalcin
Prothrombin F1 peptide
Uronic acid-rich protein
Glycosaminoglycans

In the more common calcium stone former (approximately 70% of all kidney stones), the situation is more complicated. The urine of most *normal* people is supersaturated with respect to calcium oxalate, so in principle such stones can form in all people. However, kidney stones form only in a small percentage of people with supersaturated urine, probably owing to the presence of urine inhibitors of crystallization. Some individuals may form stones primarily because of a lower than normal concentration of a urine inhibitor. Some urinary inhibitors have been identified and include both organic and inorganic substances (Table 2). Urinary citrate is an example of a clinically important inhibitor. Because citrate forms a soluble complex with calcium, low urinary citrate excretion is equivalent to increasing urinary levels of calcium [14]. An imbalance between SS and urine inhibitors is necessary for crystal nucleation. It is important to remember that any urine abnormality involving SS, urine inhibitors, or both may be the result of a *systemic disease*. For example, calcium urolithiasis may be the result of primary hyperparathyroidism, sarcoidosis, vitamin D excess, hyperthyroidism, immobilization, enteric hyperoxaluria, primary hyperoxaluria, or dehydrating bowel disease. Low citrate is another example, and may result from conditions such as distal renal tubular acidosis or chronic diarrhea syndrome.

Essential Evaluation

The end result of a metabolic evaluation may commit the patient to a treatment regimen, including dietary modifications and medication, for the rest of their life. Yet some patients will never form a stone again [23]. Therefore, it is essential to adjust the extent of the metabolic evaluation to the patient's individual circumstances, or in other words, "The punishment must fit the crime."

All stone-forming patients should have a basic evaluation as suggested in Table 3. *The history and physical examination* remain an integral part of the evaluation. Questions to be addressed include: previous episodes of urinary tract infection and stone or gravel passage; any stone analysis should be noted; family history should include specific questions about gout, cystinuria, and renal tubular acido-

TABLE 3. Essential evaluation for all stone patients

History and physical
Medical risk factors
Urinary tract infections
Previous stone events and stone analysis
Family history
Inflammatory bowel disease
Bowel surgery
Medication
Environmental risk factors
Fluid intake and diet
Occupation
Immobilization
Climate
Laboratory analysis
Urinalysis and culture
Blood
Calcium (if high then PTH levels)
Phosphorous
Electrolytes
Creatinine
Uric acid
Radiological analysis
KUB, IVP, or noncontrast CT
Stone analysis

sis or calcium urolithiasis. Some medication can increase the risk of stone formation. For example, human immunodeficiency virus (HIV) patients treated with Indinavir have an incidence of renal colic and urolithiasis of between 9.3% and 13.1% [24]. Premature infants receiving long-term furosemide therapy may develop nephrocalcinosis or nephrolithiasis, or both [25]. Systemic diseases such as hyperparathyroidism, hyperthyroidism, sarcoidosis, distal renal tubular acidosis (RTA), and myeloproliferative disorders should be recognized. Enteric hyperoxaluria can occur in Crohn's disease and other malabsorptive conditions, as well as following ileocecal resection and jejunoileal bypass [26]. Total colectomy and ileostomy are associated with increased risk of uric acid stones due to loss of water and bicarbonate in the stool [27, 28]. Environmental risk factors such as occupation, climate, and immobilization need to be considered. Dietary history should include questions concerning fluid intake, dietary supplements, and dietary indiscretion with regard to foods high in calcium, oxalate, and purines.

A *radiological examination* of the kidney, ureter, and bladder (KUB) and intravenous urography or noncontrast computerized tomography (CT) should be performed for every patient unless contraindicated. A comparison of previous films, if available, with new ones is useful. Spiral CT may also be advantageous in predicting the chemical composition of the stone [29, 30].

Stone analysis is a major first step in the evaluation of all patients. Every effort should be made to collect stone material in all patients, including patients treated with shock wave lithotripsy (SWL). On discharge, we should provide such patients with collecting devices in order to preserve any passed gravel for analysis.

Laboratory examinations include urinalysis and urine culture, serum calcium, phosphorous, uric acid, electrolytes, and creatinine concentrations. Patients should undergo parathyroid hormone essay *only* if hypercalcemia or high-normal serum calcium is found. If the stone composition is unknown, a qualitative cystine screening should be obtained.

The Single-Stone Former

Patients who present after the spontaneous passage of a single stone, or more than one stone with very long periods between episodes, are frequently encountered. Some authors would recommend an extensive metabolic evaluation for such patients because of the relatively high recurrence rate and the possibility that the initial stone event may be a harbinger of an underlying multisystem disorder [31, 32]. Others have suggested the consideration of different risk factors in order to identify patients who need further evaluation [3, 32, 33] (Table 4). Children, patients with stones composed of cystine and uric acid, patients who required surgical procedures for stone removal, patients with multiple stones or nephrocalcinosis, patients with a solitary kidney, and patients with a positive family history should probably be evaluated.

By exclusion, single-stone formers with an uneventful clinical course and without any risk factor need only the essential elements of the evaluation. The issue of further evaluation and its implications (i.e., dietary measures, long-term medication) should be discussed with the patient. Those who choose to undergo metabolic evaluation should do so even if presenting as an uncomplicated first-time stone former. However, metabolic evaluation is not helpful in predicting which patients will develop a recurrence, as patients who present after the first stone have the same pattern of metabolic disorders as patients with multiple stones [34].

TABLE 4. High-risk single-stone former

Children
Cystine and uric acid stones
Nonpure struvite stones
Multiple stones
Nephrocalcinosis
Solitary kidney
Stones requiring surgical removal

Metabolic Evaluation

Modern stone preventive measures can reduce the stone recurrence rates significantly. Medical treatment is usually not appropriate without a metabolic evaluation directing the treatment choice and the patient's follow-up. With an extensive metabolic evaluation, a metabolic or environmental etiology of nephrolithiasis can be identified in up to 97% of patients [35].

The cornerstone of metabolic evaluation is the collection of the patient's urine over a period of time. A number of protocols have been described for the metabolic evaluation of patients with recurrent stone disease or of high-risk patients. The protocols differ from one another with regard to the period of urine collection (part of the day or 24h), one or more urine collections, and provocative tests applied in some protocols that identify classifications of hypercalciuria by oral calcium deprivation and loading, or acid–loading tests for the diagnosis of RTA.

An ambulatory 24-h urine collection has been shown to be as effective as an inpatient evaluation in detecting metabolic abnormalities, and has been studied extensively [2]. Urine is collected while the patient is eating a normal diet and taking their usual medication for indications other than stone disease. Drugs prescribed for stone disease, as well as vitamin supplements, should be stopped 5 days before urine collection. It is advisable to postpone complete diagnostic evaluation for at least 1 month after the resolution of ureteral obstruction or infection, or after stone removal procedures [32]. Urine is assessed for volume and pH, and for calcium, phosphate, sodium, potassium, uric acid, magnesium, oxalate, citrate, and creatinine content (Table 5). Urinary creatinine excretion is measured to assess the adequacy of urine collection (men, 20–25mg/kg/24h; women, 15–20mg/kg/24h). SS values for specific salts are calculated using computer programs such as Equil [36].

A 24-h urine collection is most commonly used, although other periods of time have been described, such as the 16-h daytime collection reported by Tiselius [37]. As expected, repeated urine collections yield a higher diagnostic accuracy than a single collection. For example, Yagisawa et al. [38] were able to identify hypercalciuria in 47% vs. 35% of patients with two 24-h urine collections vs. one collection ($P < 0.001$). Our policy is to acquire a minimum of two random 24-h urine collections in order to correct for possible measurements or collection errors that may occur in one of the samples.

To further differentiate hypercalciuria into different subtypes, Pak et al. [39] described a method in which two 24-h urine samples from patients on a random diet are collected initially. Another 24-h urine sample is collected after 1 week of adherence to a diet restricted in calcium (400mg/day) and sodium (100mEq/day), followed by an oral calcium load test. The rationale behind Pak's protocol is the need to differentiate between the various mechanisms causing hypercalciuria. However, the issue is controversial and is reviewed further below.

Two broad theories exist about the pathogenesis of hypercalciuria. In 1974, Pak et al. [39] suggested that hypercalciuria was heterogeneous in origin and that

TABLE 5. Recurrent stone former and high-risk single-stone former metabolic evaluation

Essential evaluation as detailed plus: 24-h urine-2 samples	24-h urine reference values
Volume	>2000 cc
pH	Abnormal in: RTA >6.5, uric acid stones <5.5
Creatinine	Women: 15–20/mg/kg/24-h
	Men: 20–25/mg/kg/24-h
Calcium	Women: <250 mg/24-h
	Men: <300 mg/24-h
	<4 mg/kg/24-h for both sexes
	<140 mg calcium/g creatinine
Phosphate	500–1100 mEq/day
Potassium	25–125 mEq/day
Sodium	<200 mEq/day
Uric acid	Women <750 mg/24-h
	Men <800 mg/24-h
Oxalate	<45 mg/24-h
Citrate	>320 mg/24-h
Magnesium	>50 mg/24-h
Repeat 24-h urine annually and when diet or medication change	

three types exist: absorptive hypercalciuria, renal hypercalciuria, and resorptive hypercalciuria. Absorptive hypercalciuria was further divided into two types: type I, in which urine calcium levels are >200 mg/day during both low and high dietary calcium intake, and type II, in which hypercalciuria occurs only during high calcium intake. Coe and co-workers [40–42] maintain that such a distinction has no clinical relevance, and further that the above classification represents a spectrum of patients with the same pathogenesis (i.e., a marked increase in the fraction of dietary calcium absorbed and lost in the urine). Increased intestinal calcium absorption occurs but is not always sufficient to compensate for urinary losses, and thus the calcium balance is negative in more than half of such patients. A negative calcium balance can lead to reduced bone density in some patients, which can be exacerbated by a low-calcium diet. According to Pak, selective medical treatment adjusted to the different subclassifications of hypercalciuria is preferable. However, there is lack of conclusive experimental verification for this hypothesis [43], and there are some practical limitations to Pak's protocol which will be reviewed in the sections on treatment. Coe's unified approach maintains that calcium load studies provide no additional clinically relevant data. In our view, differentiating among the various forms of hypercalciuria should be reserved for research settings.

Follow-Up 24-h Urine Collections

The importance of repeated 24-h urine collections during follow-up *cannot* be overemphasized. Follow-up 24-h urine samples are the major way of assessing the effectiveness of the medical treatments recommended, as well as patient compliance. The 24-h urine collection should be repeated annually, and also after any change in diet or medication, or increased stone activity.

Medical Treatment

Medical treatment for stone disease is mainly intended to prevent stone recurrence and sometimes to dissolve an existing stone. Some of the measures are *nonspecific*, and are recommended for all stone-forming patients regardless of the underlying etiology. *Specific* treatments are directed by the stone etiology.

Nonspecific Treatment

Increased fluid intake increases urine output and lowers the concentration of solutes involved in stone formation. Historical data strongly suggest that hydration is effective in preventing stone formation [1]. A prospective study in which settlers in one desert town were systematically educated on their arrival to the need for a high fluid intake, while those arriving in a similar town were given no specific advice, showed that those given advice on fluid intake had a 10-fold lower incidence of urolithiasis [44]. Coe and co-workers [34] identified failure to increase urinary output as the most important factor that predicts stone recurrence. A low urine volume must be considered as a real risk factor, both for the onset of stone disease and for stone relapse [45]. Beverages other than water have also been shown to have a protective effect. Curhan et al. [46] showed a positive benefit from coffee, tea, and wine. Wabner and Pak [47] reported the beneficial effects of orange juice consumption. In contrast, grapefruit juice had an adverse effect [48]. There is a consensus that an oral fluid intake that will produce at least 2000 ml per day is a minimum hydration goal for stone patients [1].

Dietary Treatment

Calcium

An abnormally efficient intestinal absorption of dietary calcium is well known in idiopathic hypercalciuria [40]. Dietary calcium restriction can decrease urinary calcium excretion, especially in patients with hypercalciuria, and thus low-calcium diets have long enjoyed popularity. However, a low-calcium diet may increase the intestinal absorption of oxalate, and thereby reduce the effectiveness of this therapy [49]. Furthermore, bone mineral is found to be abnormally labile in patients with idiopathic hypercalciuria. Bone mineral density tends to be below normal in the majority of stone-forming patients, and some hypercalciuric patients lose bone mineral when placed on a low-calcium diet [50, 51]. Finally, in Curhan's study [46] of the relation between dietary calcium intake and the risk of symptomatic kidney stones in a cohort of 45 629 men, an inverse relationship was found between the intake of dietary calcium and the risk of kidney stones. The incidence of symptomatic kidney stones was lower by almost 50% in men with the highest calcium intake. Leonetti et al. [52] recently reported similar results supporting Curhan's study showing that a group of stone-formers had a significantly lower daily intake of calcium when compared with healthy controls (794 mg/day vs. 943 mg/day). Therefore, dietary calcium restriction is not advisable and may even be potentially harmful. A daily calcium intake of 800–1000 mg (two servings of dairy products a day) is considered adequate for calcium urolithiasis patients.

Sodium

A high sodium intake and excretion inhibits tubular reabsorption of calcium, thus increasing calcium excretion. A significant reduction in urinary calcium has been demonstrated in hypercalciuric patients after dietary sodium restriction [53]. It is reasonable, therefore, to advise calcium stone patients to avoid a high salt intake. In hypercalciuric patients treated with thiazides, a high salt intake has been shown to attenuate the hypocalciuric effect of the drug. Therefore, sodium restriction is advised for these patients [54]. Sodium excretion in the urine equals dietary consumption and should be checked in each 24-h urine sample, especially if thiazides have been prescribed. Oral intake should be limited to 100 mEq (2300 mg diet) daily.

Oxalate

A small increase in urinary oxalate excretion affects calcium oxalate SS to a larger extent than a similar increase in calcium excretion. Although most of the oxalate excreted in the urine is endogenously produced as an end product of metabolism, a mild degree of hyperoxaluria is common in stone-formers. This is secondary to increased oxalate absorption from the gastrointestinal tract [40]. Therefore, patients with mild hyperoxaluria may benefit from a low oxalate diet, avoiding foods such as spinach, rhubarb, beets, nuts, chocolate, tea, wheat bran, and strawberries [55].

Protein

Epidemiological studies showing a correlation between affluence and nephro-lithiasis implicated a diet rich in animal proteins as a risk factor for calcium nephrolithiasis and uric acid stones [56]. A high dietary protein intake is associ-ated with increased calcium excretion in healthy subjects as well as in patients

TABLE 6. Nonspecific treatment recommendations

Increase fluid intake to achieve urine output of 2 l/24-h
Limit calcium to 800–1000 mg/day (2 servings of dairy products/day)
Reduce salt intake to <100 mEq/day (no salting of food, no fast food)
Reduce protein intake (less then 12 oz of fish/beef/poultry)

with kidney stones. Further, the mild metabolic acidosis resulting from excessive protein intake might stimulate bone resorption, with a secondary increase in calcium excretion and hypocitraturia. Oxaluria and uricosuria are also associated with a high protein diet [57]. Although studies of low protein diets are not consistent in showing a beneficial effect, a decrease in dietary protein is advised for all stone patients (less then 12 oz of fish/beef/poultry per day).

In summary, for most stone-forming patients, conservative measures that include an increase in fluid intake and the elimination of dietary excesses of calcium, sodium, oxalate, and protein are advisable (Table 6). A common initial approach is to try and alter these factors before resorting to specific treatment protocols [58]. The effects of such measures have been referred to as the "stone clinic effect." In a study by Hosking et al. [59], 58% of patients (including single and recurrent stone formers) treated conservatively showed no evidence of new stone formation during a mean follow-up of >5 years. Finally, patients should be made aware that abrupt changes in fluid or sodium intake may be associated with side effects such as bloating or salt craving, respective, which resolve spontaneously with time.

Specific Treatment

Patients undergoing a metabolic evaluation will often have more than one metabolic risk factor. For example, Levy et al. [2] reported that among 1270 patients with recurrent nephrolithiasis, 41.3% were diagnosed with a single abnormality, whereas 58.7% had multiple diagnoses. All identified abnormalities should be treated. However, for simplicity we will discuss the major metabolic abnormalities separately. A general outline of the evaluation and treatment of these abnormalities is shown in Fig. 2 and will be considered in detail below.

Idiopathic Hypercalciuria

Idiopathic hypercalciuria (IH) is diagnosed in more than half of all patients with calcium oxalate stones. IH affects both sexes equally and often occurs in successive generations. There is evidence to support a complex (autosomal dominant) genetic origin for this disorder [41]. Hypercalciuria is defined as the excretion of over 300 mg/24 h for a man, over 250 mg/24 h for a woman, over 4 mg/kg body weight per 24-h for either sex, or over 140 mg/gm of creatinine. Patients with IH

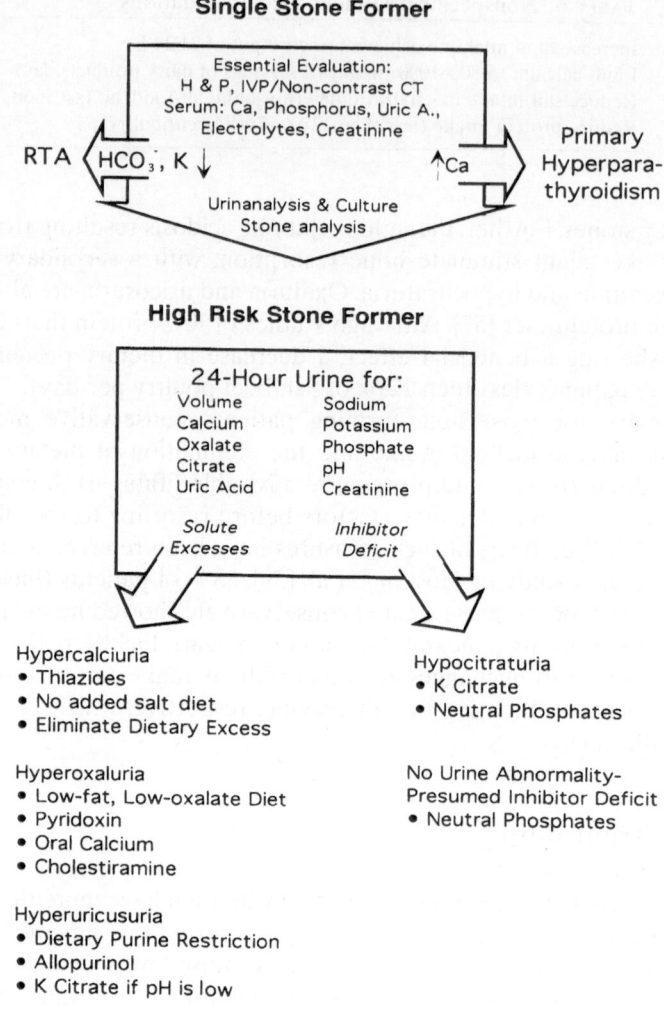

Single Stone Former

Essential Evaluation:
H & P, IVP/Non-contrast CT
Serum: Ca, Phosphorus, Uric A.,
Electrolytes, Creatinine

RTA HCO_3^-, K ↓

↑Ca Primary Hyperpara-thyroidism

Urinanalysis & Culture
Stone analysis

High Risk Stone Former

24-Hour Urine for:
Volume   Sodium
Calcium   Potassium
Oxalate   Phosphate
Citrate   pH
Uric Acid   Creatinine

Solute   Inhibitor
Excesses   Deficit

Hypercalciuria
• Thiazides
• No added salt diet
• Eliminate Dietary Excess

Hypocitraturia
• K Citrate
• Neutral Phosphates

Hyperoxaluria
• Low-fat, Low-oxalate Diet
• Pyridoxin
• Oral Calcium
• Cholestiramine

No Urine Abnormality-
Presumed Inhibitor Deficit
• Neutral Phosphates

Hyperuricusuria
• Dietary Purine Restriction
• Allopurinol
• K Citrate if pH is low

FIG. 2. Evaluation and specific treatment options for calcium stone formers

have, by definition, normal serum calcium levels and lack a definable disorder that would cause the observed elevation of urine calcium, such as RTA, sarcoidosis, hyperthyroidism, or immobilization. These disorders, as well as primary hyperparathyroidism, account for less than 10% of all calcium oxalate renal stones and will not be discussed here.

The hypothesized pathogenesis of IH can affect the choice of treatment. Dividing hypercalciuric patients into subgroups by suggesting different etiological mechanisms would be appropriate only if such distinctions would influence treatment. Thus, if the primary mechanism was believed to be intestinal overabsorption, then a low calcium diet, or drugs that reduce calcium absorption, such as cellulose phosphate, would be appropriate for this IH subgroup. However, a low calcium diet has been associated with reduced bone mineral levels and negative calcium balance [41, 50, 51], and the benefits of cellulose phosphate are doubtful [7]. Therefore, thiazide therapy is the best currently available treatment for this group of patients. For patients subclassified as having renal hypercalciuria, thiazides, which act to increase tubular reabsorption of calcium, are the treatment of choice [43]. So in practice, most hypercalciuric patients, regardless of their subgroup, will benefit from thiazide therapy.

Another problem with the structured specific approach for subgroups of hypercalciuria is that patients with hypercalciuria cannot easily be characterized into specific diagnostic groups. Recently, even Pak [60], who was the proponent of the selective approach, stated that, "There is currently no firm evidence that the selective treatments are more effective in inhibiting calcium oxalate stone formation than drugs that are applied non-selectively," and suggested that "noncomplicated" calcium stone-formers with hypercalciuria should be treated with a combination of thiazides and potassium citrate [61]. Potassium citrate helps prevent hypokalemia and hypocitraturia secondary to thiazide therapy. Therefore, thiazides have emerged as the main contemporary therapy for most IH patients [42].

Thiazides act directly on the kidney to reduce urinary calcium excretion. In addition, thiazides may cause an apparent shunting of absorbed dietary calcium into bone and reduce bone fractures by promoting a positive calcium balance [50]. Thiazide therapy is also the best-studied treatment intervention for hypercalciuric stone-formers. Although double-blind prospective studies with a limited follow-up of 1 or 2 years failed to show the effectiveness of thiazide therapy, three studies conducted over 3 years showed a significantly lower relapse rate by the third year [5, 9, 62]. Therefore, treatment of patients with thiazides should probably be planned for at least 3 years in order to achieve significant results. Optional treatment regimes that have been studied include:

1. chlorthalidone (Hygroton), 12.5–25 mg qd, up to a maximum of 100 mg qd;
2. hydrochlorothiazide (HCTZ, Esidrex, Hydrodiuril, Oretic, Microzide), 25–50 mg bid;
3. hydrochlorothiazide 50 mg with Amiloride 5 mg (moduretic), $\frac{1}{2}$ tablet bid;
4. indapamide (Lozol), 2.5 mg qd.

Patients should be advised to keep to a low-salt diet <100 mEq/day (no salting of food, and avoiding fast food) because of the negative effect of a high salt intake on thiazide efficacy. Side effects are generally mild but may occur in about 30%–50% of patients. Patients should be monitored for hypokalemia which can be corrected with potassium citrate or a potassium-sparing diuretic such as Amiloride (Midamor); 5 mg 1–3 qd. Side effects that are more common include lassitude and sleepiness. In addition, decreased libido, hypercholesteremia, and hyperuricosemia may occur.

Cellulose phosphate (Calcibind) is an oral calcium-binding resin that is taken with meals. It is effective in reducing gastrointestinal absorption of calcium.

However, it has not been shown to be effective in reducing stone formation or calcium oxalate SS in a controlled study, perhaps because it can produce secondary hyperoxaluria by making more oxalate available for absorption [63]. Some authors have used cellulose sodium phosphate in cases of documented type I absorptive hypercalciuria [22, 43]. Side effects may include nausea and diarrhea. In addition, when used in patients with normal calcium absorption, it may cause a negative calcium balance, raising the possibility of future bone disease. The resin may also cause hypomagnesemia by binding magnesium in the gut [40, 41]. In our view, cellulose phosphate is rarely, if ever, indicated in the management of patients with IH.

Orthophosphates are salts of sodium or potassium phosphate that act by decreasing urinary excretion of calcium, binding calcium in the intestinal tract, and increasing urinary inhibitor activity, probably due to stimulated renal excretion of pyrophosphate and citrate [54]. In one study, when given at an oral dose of 1500 mg per day in three to four divided doses, orthophosphates were as effective as thiazide diuretics [64]. However, in the only placebo-controlled trial reported, no effect of potassium acid phosphate therapy on stone recurrence was found [65]. That study was criticized for using acidic salt, whereas neutral phosphates reduce urinary calcium excretion more effectively. Current indications for the use of orthophosphates include IH patients who have not responded to more specific types of therapy, or who could not tolerate the thiazides. In addition, calcium oxalate stone-formers whose metabolic evaluation has failed to reveal any abnormality, and who thus may have low urine inhibitor activity, may also benefit from orthophosphate treatment. The preparations available are Neutra-Phos (one capsule or packet qid) and K-Phos neutral (250 mg, 1–2 tablets tid/qid). Orthophosphate can cause diarrhea, but this usually subsides after the first few weeks of therapy. The treatment may be associated with soft-tissue calcification in patients with renal insufficiency, but this is very rare.

Hyperuricosuria in Calcium Stone-Formers

Hyperuricosuria is defined as a daily urinary excretion above 800 mg and 750 mg for men and women, respectively. Hyperuricosuria is associated with uric acid stones, but more interestingly, this condition is found in 10%–26% of calcium stone-formers [40]. Possible mechanisms linking uric acid and calcium oxalate crystallization include heterogeneous nucleation of calcium oxalate by uric acid or its salts, and/or reduction (by binding) of naturally occurring urinary inhibitors [66]. Most hyperuricosuric calcium oxalate stone-formers have normal serum uric acid levels and often a urinary pH greater than 5.5. Hyperuricosuria generally results from increased dietary purine intake derived from meat, poultry, and fish. Dietary purine restriction seems a logical first step in treatment. However, there is no published data to support its use. Rough guidelines for such a diet have been suggested by Coe [67]: "moderate your diets; keep the total for a day of meat and poultry and of fish at one-half pound, or two-thirds pound (10–12 oz), and make the difference with breads or grains." If diet fails, medication should be administered.

Allopurinol (Zyloprim, Purinol) has been demonstrated (in a placebo-controlled randomized clinical trial in calcium oxalate stone-formers with normocalcemia and hyperuricosuria) to be effective in reducing stone recurrence [68]. The preferred dose is 100 mg tablets, 1–2 qd. Adverse effects of Allopurinol include gastrointestinal disturbances, rash, and the elevation of liver enzymes.

Hyperoxaluria

Hyperoxaluria is defined as a urinary oxalate excretion in excess of 45 mg/day for either sex. Although oxalate occurs in a majority of kidney stones, most stone-formers have normal oxalate excretion rates of between 20 and 40 mg/24 h [41]. Excessive urinary oxalate originates either from enhanced intestinal absorption, so-called "enteric hyperoxaluria," or from enhanced endogenous production (which usually accounts for most excreted urinary oxalate).

Endogenous oxalate overproduction is rare and results from a congenital condition termed "primary hyperoxaluria." There are two types of hereditary autosomal recessive hyperoxaluria. In the more common type I (1 : 120 000 live births), reduced activity of hepatic peroxisomal alanine-glyoxylate aminotransferase (AGT) increases the availability of glyoxylate, which is converted to oxalic acid. In type II, excretion of L-glyceric acid is increased. Recently, a third type (nontype-1, nontype-2) of hyperoxaluria has been described. Urine oxalate levels in the hereditary forms are typically very high: between 135 and 270 mg/day. Patients with congenital hyperoxaluria begin stone formation in early childhood, and later may develop nephrocalcinosis, accumulation of insoluble oxalate through the body (oxalosis), or tubulointerstitial nephropathy. About half will progress to end-stage renal disease by the age of 15 [69].

Pyridoxine at dosages of 2–15 mg/kg/day has been shown to reduce oxalate excretion to normal levels in about 20% of cases, and to reduce oxalate levels to some extent in about one-third of patients with type I disease [70]. Other treatment modalities include high fluid intake supported by calcium oxalate crystallization inhibitors, i.e., potassium citrate, 150 mg/kg/day, or orthophosphate, 30 mg/kg/day. Thiazide therapy may also be added [70].

Enteric hyperoxaluria can occur in patients with intestinal fat malabsorption from any cause. Examples include inflammatory bowel disease, celiac sprue, pancreatic insufficiency, and jejunoileal bypass. Long-chain fatty acids and bile acids increase colonic permeability to oxalate and bind calcium, thus freeing oxalate for absorption [71]. Since calcium absorption is severely decreased, these patients typically have very low urinary calcium excretion (i.e., <100 mg/day). Since oxalate absorption occurs in the large intestine, an intact colon is necessary for enteric hyperoxaluria to occur [72]. Treatment strategies include conservative dietary measures (low fat, low oxalate) combined with, or followed by, medication that reduces oxalate absorption, as described below.

Oral calcium supplements such as Tums can bind free oxalate and limit absorption. One to two grams with each meal is the recommended dose [73].

Cholestyramine (Questran), 4 g, 1–6 times/day with meals, is a nonabsorbable resin that binds fatty acids, bile acids, and oxalate, thus reducing the available oxalate. It is a useful drug because it helps to reduce diarrhea, which is a major problem for many malabsorption patients. Cholestyramine can cause vitamin K depletion, and therefore prothrombin time should be measured every 6 months. Some patients with malabsorptive syndromes may exhibit hypomagnesiuria, which can be corrected with oral magnesium supplements.

Hypocitraturia

Low urinary citrate can raise the risk of stones because citrate is a strong calcium-binding molecule which forms a soluble salt, and which may also act as an inhibitor of crystallization. Hypocitraturia is defined as a 24-h excretion of citrate of less than 320 mg and is found in 15%–60% of stone-formers, often in combination with other metabolic abnormalities. The most important regulator of citrate reabsorption is systemic acid–base status. Acidosis decreases renal citrate excretion, while alkalosis has the opposite effect. Hypokalemia, a high animal protein diet, and urinary tract infection can also lower urinary citrate levels. Hypocitraturia is invariably found in patients with distal RTA (who typically have profoundly low citrate levels, i.e., <50 mg/day), and is also associated with chronic diarrhea states and diuretic-induced hypokalemia. However, in most cases no underlying cause is found [40, 41, 54]. Correcting the remediable causes of hypocitraturia is the first treatment step. Administrating a base such as potassium bicarbonate or potassium citrate will increase citrate excretion. Sodium bases may increase urinary calcium excretion and thus offset the benefits of increased urinary citrate. In prospective randomized clinical trials, potassium citrate has been shown to significantly decrease stone recurrence [74]. Recently, potassium citrate has been shown to be effective in preventing stone recurrence regardless of stone composition, metabolic abnormalities, or stone-free status [75]. A new drug (K-Mag), which is a combination of potassium citrate and magnesium, has been shown in a placebo-controlled randomized trial to be effective in inhibiting calcium stone formation [61]. Preparations are available in tablet form (UroCit K), or in solution (PolyCitra-K syrup, PolyCitra-K crystals, K Lyte). The initial dose should be 20–30 mEq bid.

Uric Acid Stones

Uric acid SS is driven by three factors: acidic urine, decreased urine volume, and hyperuricosuria. Urine pH is the major determinant of uric acid SS [71]. Urine pH changes have a greater impact on uric acid stone formation than changes in uric acid excretion. An increase in urine pH from 5 to 6.5 will increase the solubility of uric acid by a factor of 10 [76]. The mean pH of patients who form uric acid stones is 5.5 ± 0.4, compared with 6 ± 0.4 in calcium oxalate stone formers [41]. Uric acid is the major end-product of purine metabolism, with approximately one-half originating from the diet. Either increased purine ingestion or endogenous uric acid over production may increase the amount of uric acid that must be excreted daily. Although most patients with uric acid stones excrete more than 750 mg/day of uric acid, idiopathic (sporadic or familial) uric acid stone patients have normal levels of urine and serum uric acid. However, like most uric acid stone formers, they excrete less ammonia, and therefore have markedly acidic urine [40]. The treatment of uric acid stones is unique in that the goals of the treatment are the dissolution of existing stones as well as the prevention of stone recurrence. Patients are advised to increase fluid intake and consume a low-purine diet. Alkalinization is aimed at increasing urinary pH above pH 5.5, and preferably between 6 and 6.5 [41, 43]. Citrate may be preferred over bicarbonate because it requires less frequent doses. The usual dose to maintain a pH of 6.5 is 30–60 mEq per day in two divided doses (available preparations have been discussed previously). Allopurinol is recommended for patients with hyperuricemia, patients with uric acid excretion greater than 1000 mg/day, before chemotherapy in myeloproliferative diseases, and for stone dissolution. The preferred dose is 100–200 mg/day.

Cystine Stones

Cystinuria is a rare, but important, hereditary autosomal recessive disease in which there is a tubular defect of dibasic amino acid transport. Large amounts of cystine, ornithine, lysine, and arginine ("COLA") are excreted into the urine due to an inability to reabsorb them in the proximal tubule of the kidney. Cystine excretion, leading to the formation of cystine calculi, is the only clinically significant consequence of cystinuria. Functionally, a patient who excretes more than 250 mg cystine per g creatinine in a 24-h urine collection (normal values are 30–50 mg/day) is defined as having cystinuria; hexagonal crystals found upon microscopic examination of urinary sediment are diagnostic, but are found in only 17%–26% of patients [77, 78]. Cystine stones are relatively infrequent, and account for approximately 1% of all kidney stones (about 6% in the pediatric population), but cystinuria is one of the more frequent inherited disorders, with an incidence of 1/2500 in Israeli Jews and 1/15000 in the United States [79]. Stones of mixed composition are sometimes present in cystinuric patients and may represent associated metabolic abnormalities [76]. The genetics of cystinuria are complex, and the actual biochemical defects in cell transport are not yet well understood.

Cystinurics are segregated into three subtypes according to differences in intestinal transport in the homozygotes and the urinary phenotype of heterozygotes. Type I is inherited in an autosomal recessive manner and is the most common type, accounting for approximately two-thirds of all homozygous patients. Type I homozygotes have no intestinal mucosa cystine transport, while heterozygotes have a normal urine cystine excretion. Types II and III have an incomplete recessive transmission with varying degrees of intestinal mucosa transport defect and an elevated urinary excretion of cystine in the heterozygotes [78]. Nephrolithiasis in cystinuric patients usually presents by the fourth decade (average age of presentation is 22), although later presentations have been recorded. The treatment of cystinuria is designed to reduce the SS of cystine. Increasing the urinary volume to more than 2.5 l/day is the first approach. The second step in the therapy takes advantage of the effect of pH on cystine solubility. Cystine solubility is pH-dependent, with gradually increasing solubility to pH 7.5, and rapidly increasing solubility above pH 7.5. Increasing urine pH above 7.5 will increase cystine solubility, but this pH is often difficult to maintain on a chronic basis, and may place the patient at a risk of forming apatite stones. Therefore, the desired pH range is between 7 and 7.5. [40, 71, 76]. Potassium citrate is most commonly used for alkalinization at a dose of 30 mEq of base four times daily.

Methionine is the precursor of cystine stones, and dietary restriction has been the recommended treatment. However, such diets require severe protein restriction and are unpalatable, leading to poor patient compliance. A more practical approach would be to adhere to the general dietary measures discussed previously, especially sodium restriction. Studies have shown that sodium restriction reduces urinary cystine excretion [80]. When conservative measures are ineffective α-mercaptopropionylglycine (α-MPG) or D-penicillamine can be used. Both drugs act by forming disulfide complexes with cysteine, so instead of two cysteine molecules combining to form cystine, a cysteine molecule combines with the drug to form a soluble drug–cysteine complex. D-penicillamine (Cuprimine, Depen) comes in 125 and 250 capsules. Each gram of D-penicillamine can be expected to dissolve 300 mg cystine [79]. Therefore, it is usually administered at 125–250 mg qid and titrated to obtain urinary concentrations of cystine below 300 mg/l. Side effects are common, and include skin rash, gastrointestinal upset, athralgia, fever, agranulocytosis, loss of taste and smell, proteinuria, and nephritic syndrome. Over 50% of patients are unable to tolerate doses sufficient to lower cystine levels [78, 79]. α-MPG (Thiola, Tiopronin) appears to be better tolerated than D-penicillamine, and side effects are similar but less severe. The usual dose of Thiola is 10–30 mg/kg/day divided into three or four doses (100-mg tablets). Finally, the angiotensin-converting enzyme inhibitor captopril, which contains a thiol group similar to α-MPG and D-penicillamine, has recently been shown to decrease urinary cystine at doses of 75–100 mg/day in some affected patients. However, its clinical value in lowering the new stone formation has yet to be determined [81].

Struvite Stones

Struvite stones are composed of mixtures of magnesium, ammonium, phosphate, and carbonate apatite. Unlike other stones discussed in this chapter, struvite stones do not result from a metabolic abnormality but are a result of urinary tract infection associated with urease-producing bacteria. Therefore, struvite stones are often referred to as "infection stones." Bacterial urease hydrolyzes urea to form ammonia and carbon dioxide. Consumption of hydrogen ions in the process increases urine pH. The presence of ammonia and a urine pH greater than 7.2 are required for struvite stone formation [76]. Propagation of struvite stone formation may be enhanced by the adhesion of struvite crystals to the urothelium, specifically to the charged sulfate group of the glycosaminoglycan (GAG) layer protecting the urothelium [82]. The most common organism associated with struvite calculi is *Proteus mirabilis*. Other common pathogens that frequently produce urease are *Providencia, Klebsiella, Pseudomonas,* and *Enterococci.* Although some authors have suggested that metabolic abnormalities are commonly present in patients with infected stones, others have found that stone recurrence after complete elimination of the calculi is uncommon. Different definitions of the term "infection stone," and particularly the inclusion of mixed struvite and calcium oxalate stones, may explain the contradictory results. We have found that in a group of patients with infection stones, those with pure struvite stones were significantly less likely to have metabolic abnormalities than patients who had struvite stone mixed with calcium oxalate [83]. The best treatment for struvite stones is complete stone removal and eradication of the urinary infection. Patients waiting for stone removal surgery should begin culture-specific or broad-spectrum antibiotics 2 weeks before surgery. After clearance of struvite calculi, 3 months of oral culture-specific antibiotic treatment is recommended [76]. Struvite stones tend to recur in approximately 10% of patients after complete stone removal, and in up to 85% of patients with stone remnants. High-risk patients (paralyzed patients, patients with urinary diversion, neurogenic bladder, etc.) may require long-term antibiotic prophylaxis. Acetohydroxamic acid (AHA), an inhibitor of bacterial urease, provides another alternative treatment, in conjunction with antibiotic therapy, in patients in whom surgical intervention is contraindicated or in patients with repeated infections despite stone removal [84]. AHA has been shown, in three randomized, double-blind trials, to be effective in reducing the rate of stone growth or recurrence [40]. However, AHA has significant side effects, which limit its usefulness. The side effects of AHA include gastrointestinal upset, deep venous thrombosis (DVT), and neurologic symptoms such as headache, tremulousness, loss of taste, and hallucinations. AHA also induces low-grade intravascular coagulation [85]. AHA is contraindicated in patients with serum creatinine over 2 mg/dl. AHA (Lithostat) comes in 250-mg tablets, and the starting dose is 250 mg bid.

Urine acidification, although not studied extensively, may be another way of reducing the risk of stone recurrence. Wall and Tiselius [86] studied the effects of ammonium chloride, ascorbic acid, and methenamine hippurate on urine pH in a group of 14 normal subjects. Only ammonium chloride, in daily doses of 1.5 or 3 g, significantly reduced urinary pH. Eleven patients who were treated for infected stones received long-term (24–39 months) treatment with ammonium chloride. No adverse reactions were recorded with the dosage used. Other authors have reported that gastrointestinal upset is a common side-effect of ammonium chloride and is dose-dependent [87].

References

1. Consensus conference (1988) Prevention and treatment of kidney stones. JAMA 260:977–981
2. Levy FL, Adams-Huet, Pak CYC (1995) Ambulatory evaluation of nephrolithiasis: an update of a 1980 protocol. Am J Med 98:50–59
3. Marangella M, Vitale C, Bagnis C, Bruno M, Ramello A (1999) Idiopathic calcium nephrolithiasis. Nephron 81(Suppl 1):38–44
4. Clark JY, Thompson IM, Optenberg SA (1995) Economic impact of urolithiasis in the United States. J Urol 154:2020–2024
5. Parks JH, Coe FL (1996) Pathogenesis and treatment of calcium stones. Semin Nephrol 16:398–411
6. Parks JH, Coe FL (1996) The financial effects of kidney stone prevention. Kidney Int 50:1706–1712
7. Tomson CRV (1995) Prevention of recurrent calcium stones: a rational approach. Br J Urol 76:419–424
8. Williams RE (1963) Long-term survey of 538 patients with upper urinary tract stone. Br J Urol 35:416
9. Borghi L, Meschi T, Guerra A, Noverini A (1993) Randomized prospective study of a nonthiazide diuretic, Indapamide, in preventing calcium stone recurrences. J Cardiovasc Pharmacol 22(Suppl 6):S78–S86
10. Lingeman JE (1983) Nephrolithiasis: a controllable disease. Indiana Med 17:313
11. Parks JH, Coward M, Coe FL (1997) Correspondence between stone composition and urine supersaturation in nephrolithiasis. Kidney Int 51:894–900
12. Fleisch H (1978) Inhibitors and promoters of stone formation. Kidney Int 13:361–371
13. Melnick I, Landes RR, Hoffman AA, Burch JF (1971) Magnesium therapy for recurring calcium oxalate urinary calculi. J Urol 105:119–122
14. Pak CYC, Sakhaee K, Fuller CJ (1983) Physiological and physiochemical prevention of calcium-stone formation by potassium citrate therapy. Trans Assoc Am Phys 96:294–305
15. Hess B, Nakagawa Y, Parks JH, Coe FL (1991) Molecular abnormality of Tamm–Horsfall glycoprotein in calcium oxalate nephrolithiasis. Am J Physiol 260:F569–F578
16. Asplin JR, Arsenault D, Parks JH, Coe FL, Hoyer JR (1998) Contribution of human uropontin to inhibition of calcium oxalate crystallization. Kidney Int 53:194–199
17. Asplin J, Deganello S, Nakagawa YN, Coe FL (1991) Evidence that nephrocalcin inhibits nucleation of calcium oxalate monohydrate crystals. Am J Physiol 261:F824–F830
18. Doyle IR, Marshall VR, Dawson CJ, Ryall RL (1995) Calcium oxalate crystal matrix extract: the most potent macromolecular inhibitor of crystal growth and aggregation yet tested in undiluted human urine in vitro. Urol Res 23:53–62
19. Atmani F, Khan SR (1995) Characterization of uronic-acid-rich inhibitor of calcium oxalate crystallization isolated from rat urine. Urol Res 23:95–101
20. Cao LC, Boeve ER, de Bruijn WC, Kok DJ, de Water R, Deng G, Schroder FH (1997) Glycosaminoglycans and semi-synthetic sulfated polysaccharides: an overview of their potential application in treatment of patients with urolithiasis. Urology 50:173–183
21. Pillay S, Asplin JR, Coe FL (1998) Evidence that calgranulin is produced by kidney cells and is an inhibitor of calcium oxalate crystallization. Am J Physiol 275:F255–F261
22. McDonald MW, Stoller M (1997) Urinary stone disease: a practical guide to metabolic evaluation. Geriatrics 52(5):38–40

23. Tiselius HG (1994) Investigation of single and recurrent stone formers. Miner Electrolyte Metab 20:321–327
24. Kohan AD, Armenakas NA, Fracchia JA (1999) Indinavir urolithiasis: an emerging cause of renal colic in patients with human immunodeficiency virus. J Urol 161:1765–1768
25. Cohen TD, Ehreth J, King LR, Preminger GM (1996) Pediatric urolithiasis: medical and surgical management. Urology 47:292–303
26. Cryer PE, Garber AJ, Joffsten P (1975) Renal failure after small intestinal bypass for obesity. Arch Intern Med 135:1610–1612
27. Gigax JH, Leach JR (1971) Uric acid calculi associated with ileostomy for ulcerative colitis. J Urol 105:777–779
28. Dobbins JW, Binder HJ (1976) Effect of bile salts and fatty acids on the colonic absorption of oxalate. Gastroenterology 70:1096–1100
29. Mostafavi MR, Ernst RD, Saltzman B (1998) Accurate determination of chemical composition of urinary calculi by spiral computerized tomography. J Urol 159: 673–675
30. Saw KC, McAteer JA, Monga A, Chua GT, Lingeman JE, Williams JC (2000) Helical CT of urinary calculi: Effect of stone composition, stone size, and scan collimation. Am J Roentgenol 175:329–332
31. Pak CYC (1982) Should patients with single renal stone occurrence undergo diagnostic evaluation? J Urol 127:855–858
32. Preminger GM (1989) The metabolic evaluation of patients with recurrent nephrolithiasis: a review of comprehensive and simplified approaches. J Urol 141: 760–763
33. Tiselius HG (1994) Investigation of single and recurrent stone formers. Miner Electrolyte Metab 20:321–327
34. Strauss AL, Coe FL, Parks JH (1982) Formation of a single calcium stone of renal origin: clinical and laboratory characteristics of patients. Arch Intern Med 142:504–507
35. Preminger GM (1995) Medical management of urinary calculus disease. Part 1. Pathogenesis and evaluation. AUA Update Ser 14:38
36. Werness PG, Brown CM, Smith LH, Finlayson B (1985) Equil2: a basic computer program for the calculation of urinary saturation. J Urol 134:1242–1244
37. Tiselius HG (1997) Metabolic evaluation of patients with stone disease. Urol Int 59:131–141
38. Yagisawa T, Chandhoke PS, Fan J (1999) Comparison of comprehensive and limited metabolic evaluations in the treatment of patients with recurrent calcium urolithiasis. J Urol 161:1449–1452
39. Pak CYC, Ohata M, Lawrence EC, Snyder W (1974) The hypercalciurias: courses, parathyroid functions and idiopathic criteria. J Clin Invest 54:387–400
40. Asplin JR, Favus MJ, Coe FL (1996) Nephrolithiasis. In: Brenner BM (ed) Brenner and Rector's The Kidney, 5th edn. Saunders, Philadelphia, pp 1893–1935
41. Coe FL, Parks JH, Asplin JR (1992) The pathogenesis and treatment of kidney stones. N Engl J Med 327:1141–1152
42. Coe FL, Parks JH (1977) New insights into the pathophysiology and treatment of nephrolithiasis: new research venues. J Bone Miner Res 12:522
43. Preminger GM (1995) Medical management of urinary calculus disease. Part II. Classification of metabolic disorders and selective medical treatment. AUA Update Ser 14:38

44. Frank M, de Vries A, Tikva P (1966) Prevention of urolithiasis. Arch Environ Health 13:625–630

45. Borghi L, Meschi T, Schianchi T, Briganti A, Guerra A, Allegri F, Novarini A (1999) Urine volume: stone risk factor and preventive measure. Nephron 81(Suppl 1):31–37

46. Curhan GC, Willett WC, Rimm EB, Stampeer MJ (1993) A prospective study of dietary calcium and other nutrients and the risk of symptomatic kidney stones. N Engl J Med 12:833–838

47. Wabner CL, Pak CYC (1993) Effect of orange juice consumption on urinary stone risk factors. J Urol 149:1405–1408

48. Goldfarb DS, Coe FL (1999) Beverages, diet and prevention of kidney stones. Am J Kidney Dis 33:398–400

49. Bataille P, Pruna A, Gregoire I (1983) Critical role of oxalate restriction in association with calcium restriction to decrease the probability of being a stone former: insufficient effect in idiopathic hypercalciuria. Proc Eur Dial Transplant Assoc 20:401–406

50. Coe FL, Parks JH, Favus MJ (1997) Diet and calcium: the end of an era? Ann Intern Med 126:553–555

51. Trinchieri A, Nespoli R, Ostini F, Rovera F, Zanetti G, Pisani E (1998) A study of dietary calcium and other nutrients in idiopathic renal calcium stone formers with low bone mineral content. J Urol 159:654–657

52. Leonetti F, Dussol B, Berthezene P, Thirion X, Berland Y (1998) Dietary and urinary risk factors for stones in idiopathic calcium stone formers compared with healthy subjects. Nephrol Dial Trans 13:617

53. Silver J, Rubinger D, Friedlaender MM, Popovtzer MM (1983) Sodium-dependent idiopathic hypercalciuria in renal stone formers. Lancet 2:484–486

54. Ruml LA, Pearle MS, Pak CYC (1997) Medical therapy calcium oxalate urolithiasis. Urol Clin North Am 24:117–133

55. Massey LK, Sutton RA (1993) Modification of dietary oxalate and calcium reduces urinary oxalate in hyperoxaluric patients with kidney stones. J Am Diet Assoc 93:1305–1307

56. Parivar F, Low RK, Stoller ML (1996) The influence of diet on urinary stone disease. J Urol 155:432–440

57. Breslau NA, Brinkley L, Hill K, Pak CYC (1988) Relationship of animal protein-rich diet to kidney stone formation and calcium metabolism. J Clin Endocrin Metab 66:140

58. Wilson DM (1989) Clinical and laboratory approaches for evaluation of nephrolithiasis. J Urol 141:770–774

59. Hosking DH, Erickson SB, Van Den Berg CJ, Wilson DM, Smith LH (1983) The stone clinic effect in patients with idiopathic calcium urolithiasis. J Urol 130:1115–1118

60. Pak CY (1999) Medical prevention of renal stones. Nephron 81(Suppl 1):60–65

61. Pak CYC (1997) Southwestern internal medicine conference: medical management of nephrolithiasis—a new, simplified approach for general practice. Am J Med Sci 313:215–219

62. Ettinger B, Citron JT, Livermore B, Dolman LI (1988) Chlorthalidone reduces calcium oxalate calculus recurrence but magnesium hydroxide does not. J Urol 139:679–684

63. Backman U, Danielson BG, Johansson G, Ljughall S, Wikstrom B (1980) Treatment of recurrent calcium stone formation with cellulose phosphate. J Urol 123:9–13

64. Insogna KL, Ellison AS, Burtis WJ, Sartori L, Lang RL, Broadus AE (1989) Trichloromethiazide and oral phosphate in patients with absorptive hypercalciuria. J Urol 141:269–274

65. Ettinger B (1976) Recurrent nephrolithiasis: natural history and effect of phosphate therapy. Am J Med 61:200–206
66. Seftel A, Resnick MI (1990) Metabolic evaluation of urolithiasis. Urol Clin North Am 17:159–169
67. Coe FL (1991) Commentary: Allopurinol treatment of uric-acid disorders in calcium-stone formers. J Lithotr Stone Dis 3:272
68. Ettinger B, Tang A, Citron JT et al. (1986) Randomized trial of Allopurinol in the prevention of calcium oxalate calculi. N Engl J Med 315:1386–1389
69. Cochat P (1999) Primary hyperoxaluria type I. KI 55:2533
70. Toussaint C (1998) Pyridoxine-responsive PH1: treatment. J Nephrol 11(Suppl 1):49–50
71. Bushinsky DA (1998) Nephrolithiasis. J Am Soc Nephrol 9:917–924
72. Dobbins JW, Binder HJ (1977) Importance of colon in enteric hyperoxaluria. N Engl J Med 296:298–301
73. Earnest DL, Gausher S, Admirand WH (1976) Treatment of enteric hyperoxaluria with calcium aluminum. Gastroenterology 70:881A
74. Barcelo P, Wuhl O, Servitge E, Rousaud A, Pak CYC (1993) Randomized double-blind study of potassium citrate in idiopathic hypocitraturic calcium nephrolithiasis. J Urol 150:1761–1764
75. Lee YH, Huang WC, Tsai JY et al. (1999) The efficacy of potassium citrate based medical prophylaxis for preventing upper urinary tract calculi: a midterm follow-up study. J Urol 161:1453–1457
76. Dretler SP (1998) The physiologic approach to the medical management of stone disease. Urol Clin North Am 25:613–623
77. Lee YH, Huang WC, Tsai JY et al. (1999) The efficacy of potassium citrate based medical prophylaxis for preventing upper urinary tract calculi: a midterm follow-up study. J Urol 161:1453–1457
78. Gitomer WL, Pak CYC (1996) Recent advances in the biochemical and molecular biological basis of cystinuria. J Urol 156:1907–1912
79. Gupta M, Bolton DM, Stoller ML (1995) Etiology and management of cystine lithiasis. Urology 45:344–355
80. Rutchik SD, Resnick MI (1997) Cystine calculi. Urol Clin North Am 24:163–171
81. Norman RW, Manette WA (1990) Dietary restriction of sodium as a means of reducing urinary cystine. J Urol 143:1193–1195
82. Chow GK, Streem SB (1996) Medical treatment of cystinuria: results of contemporary clinical practice. J Urol 156:1576–1578
83. Lingeman JE, Segel YI, Steele B (1995) Metabolic evaluation of infected renal lithiasis: clinical relevance. J Endourol 9:51–54
84. Wang LP, Wong HY, Griffith DP (1997) Treatment options in struvite stones. Urol Clin North Am 21:149–162
85. Rodman JS (1999) Struvite stones. Nephron 81(Suppl 1):50–59
86. Wall I, Tiselius HG (1990) Long-term acidification of urine in patients treated for infected renal stones. Urol Int 45:336–341
87. Lutzeyer W, Hering F (1986) Drug therapy of urinary calculi and prevention of recurrence. In: Schneider HJ (ed) Urolithiasis. Springer, Berlin, pp 34–41

Contemporary Management of Distal Ureteral Calculi

Matthew T. Gettman and Margaret S. Pearle

Summary. The optimal treatment for distal ureteral calculi is controversial. The vast majority of distal stones are successfully treated with ureteroscopy (URS) or shock wave lithotripsy (SWL), and the rare endourological failure is salvaged with laparoscopic or, less commonly, open ureterolithotomy. The published literature supports both URS and SWL treatment of small to moderate size distal ureteral stones. Although stone-free rates are comparable for the two modalities, patient morbidity favors SWL, while cost favors URS. Based on stone-free rates, complication rates, and patient symptoms and satisfaction, SWL using a Dornier HM3 should constitute first-line therapy for stones ≤15 mm in diameter. For newer-generation lithotripters, the advantages may be less clear and further trials are needed. For large or multiple stones, URS is the preferred treatment modality.

Key Words. Distal ureteral calculi, Ureteroscopy, Shock wave lithotripsy, Urolithiasis, Laparoscopy

Introduction

The evolution of the treatment of distal ureteral calculi is an endourological success story. Indeed, few pathological conditions in urology have been treated as successfully as the distal ureteral stone. Endourological modalities—shock wave lithotripsy (SWL) and ureteroscopy (URS)—have all but eliminated the need for open surgical techniques, and even the rare endourological failure can often be salvaged laparoscopically.

With success, however, comes controversy, and the endourological community is sharply divided into two camps: those favoring URS and those favoring SWL.

Department of Urology, University of Texas Southwestern Medical Center, 5323 Harry Hines Blvd., Dallas, TX 75390-9110, USA

Both treatment modalities are associated with high success rates and few complications. Proponents of URS cite the ready availability of equipment and the immediacy of the outcome; in contrast, advocates of SWL argue that without compromising efficacy, SWL is associated with a lower potential for serious complications and is preferred by patients because it is completely noninvasive.

In this review, we take a critical look at outcomes for the available treatment modalities for distal ureteral calculi, and offer guidelines for treatment selection.

Historical Perspectives

Minimally invasive treatment of upper urinary tract calculi originated with transurethral means of blind stone extraction using ureteral catheters or bougies to dilate the ureteral orifice and dislodge the stone [1]. Later, with the development of the cystoscope and basket extractors, stone retrieval was enhanced with the aid of fluoroscopic visualization. Finally, the development of the purpose-built ureteroscope made stone extraction and fragmentation safer and more precise under direct endoscopic vision [2]. Even older ureteroscopy series for the treatment of distal ureteral calculi, in which large-caliber ureteroscopes and primarily direct extraction methods were used, yielded success rates between 83% and 94% [3–7]. With current small-caliber, semirigid ureteroscopes and a variety of intracorporeal lithotripsy devices, access to the distal ureter and fragmentation of the stone is a near certainty, and morbidity has been substantially reduced by eliminating the need for dilation of the intramural ureter and intact stone removal. Indeed, ureteroscopic management (URS) of distal ureteral calculi has become one of the most widely practiced and highly successful procedures in urological practice.

Shockwave lithotripsy, however, introduced a completely noninvasive treatment modality for upper urinary tract calculi. Originally intended for renal and proximal ureteral calculi, SWL indications were expanded to include distal ureteral calculi only after modification of the patient support apparatus on the Dornier HM3 lithotripter (Dornier Medical Systems, Marietta, GA, USA) was introduced to allow the unimpeded passage of shock waves into the pelvis. By using a "sitting" position [8], or by extending and flattening the chair gantry [9], the shock waves could be directed through the obturator foramen or greater sciatic notch into the pelvis to the stone. The use of a Stryker frame modification of the gantry and supine positioning also allowed the stone to be approached transgluteally [10, 11].

The application of SWL to distal ureteral calculi was further limited by poor fluoroscopic visualization of the stone owing to the overlying pelvic bone. Although the early use of a ureteral stent or catheter with injected contrast improved stone targeting, the intravenous administration of contrast to opacify the ureter obviated the need for a ureteral catheter and made in situ SWL treatment of distal ureteral stones feasible [12, 13].

Treatment Options

Observation

Because the majority of distal ureteral calculi will be passed spontaneously, conservative therapy is a reasonable treatment option in selected cases. Over a 4-year period, Morse and Resnick [14] reviewed 378 patients diagnosed as having a ureteral stone, and found a spontaneous passage rate of 71% for the 274 stones located in the distal ureter at the time of presentation. Recently, Miller and Kane [15] prospectively evaluated 75 patients with ureteral stones to assess spontaneous passage rates. Among the 58 distal ureteral calculi, spontaneous passage occurred in 87.7% of cases. The time interval to spontaneous passage averaged 8.2 days for ≤2-mm stones, 14.5 days for 2–4-mm stones, and 5.5 days for ≥4-mm stones. Thus one might reasonably expect upwards of three-quarters of distal ureteral calculi to pass spontaneously within a 6-week period.

Ureteral Stent Placement

Ureteral stents have been used to facilitate spontaneous stone passage [16] by allowing temporary passive dilation of the ureter. Leventhal and colleagues prospectively evaluated 27 patients presenting with a symptomatic solitary distal ureteral stone <10 mm in diameter; 17 patients (63%) were initially managed with an internal ureteral stent, and 10 patients were treated with URS as the definitive treatment of their stone. No significant difference in mean stone size was detected between the groups (5.4 mm × 3.5 mm for the stent group versus 5.6 mm × 3.1 mm for the URS group). No ureteroscopic complications were reported. The stents were removed from the stented group approximately 2 weeks after placement, after which 83% of patients spontaneously passed their stone at a mean of 6.6 days (range 0–25 days). Spontaneous stone passage failed to occur within 2 weeks of stent removal in three patients who ultimately underwent successful URS treatment. Thus, although simple ureteral stent placement may result in spontaneous stone passage in some patients with small distal ureteral calculi, one might argue that passage of a small-caliber semirigid ureteroscope for definitive stone management is nearly as easy, and indeed preferable, to passage of a 7F ureteral stent.

Ureteroscopy

A review of contemporary ureteroscopy series (from 1990 to the present) reveals uniformly high success rates, ranging from 86% to 100%, despite a wide variety of ureteroscopes and intracorporeal lithotripsy devices (Table 1). Complication rates have improved with time as ureteroscopes have become smaller and intracorporeal lithotripsy devices have become safer; currently, the incidence of ureteral perforation is less than 4% [17–22] and the ureteral stricture rate is less than 2% [18, 19, 21].

TABLE 1. Results of ureteroscopy for distal ureteral calculi

Author	Patients (stones)	Size of ureteroscope	Modality of stone removal	Stone-free rate	Length of stay (days)	Complications	2nd procedure
Dretler [44]	149 (151)	7.2F, 9.5F	Intact, pulsed-dye laser	98.6% (149/151)	–	1% (1/149)	1% (1/149)
Dretler and Bhatta [45]	43	7.2F, 9.5F	Intact, USL, pulsed-dye laser	95.3% (41/43)	–	–	5% (2/43)
Fugelso and Neal [46]	139	7.2F, 8.5F	Pulsed-dye laser	90.6% (126/139)	–	–	–
Garvin and Clayman [47]	104 (108)	11.5F, 12.5F	Intact, pulsed-dye laser, EHL	100% (108/108)	–	0% (0/108)	0% (0/108)
Esuvaranathan et al. [48]	64	7.2F	Pulsed-dye laser	100% (64/64)	–	–	–
Kapoor et al. [36]	32 (35)	–	Intact, EHL, USL	96.7% (31/32)	1.3	6.3% (2/32)	–
Benizri et al. [49]	84	6.5F, 7.5F	Pulsed-dye laser, Alexandrite laser	94% (79/84)	–	–	1% (1/84)
Chang et al. [34]	113	8.5F, 9.5F, 11.5F	Intact, EHL	92.0% (104/113)	2.3	8.8% (10/113)	6.2% (7/113)
Anderson et al. [25]	27	6.9F, 12F, 9.4F	Intact, EHL, pulsed-dye laser	100% (27/27)	37% outpatients, 63% 2.5 days	3.7% (1/27)	4%(1/27)
Delivcliotis et al. [17]	50	11.5F	Intact, EHL, USL, lithoclast	100% (50/50)	–	4% (2/50)	0% (0/50)
Jung et al. [22]	156	6.5F	Alexandrite laser	94.5% (148/156)	–	0% (0/156)	5% (8/156)
Yiu et al. [50]	37	7F	Holmium:YAG laser	92%	–	5.4% (2/37)	0% (0/37)
Netto et al. [21]	322	11.5F	Basket	98.1% (316/322)	0.15	4.3% (14/322)	0% (0/322)
Netto et al. [21]	161	11.5F	USL	95.6% (154/161)	2.1	16.1% (26/161)	1% (1/161)
Harmon et al. [51]	109	6F, 8.5F, 11.5F	Intact, EHL, USL, impactor	97% (106/109)	–	–	–
Eden et al. [20]	134	7F, 9.5F, 11.5F	Lithoclast	89.5% (120/134)	1.1	2.2% (3/134)	6.0% (8/134)
Kupeli et al. [52]	430	9.5%.12F	EHL, USL, lithoclast	91.9% (395/430)	–	12.6% (54/430)	22.3% (96/430)
Yip et al. [53]	34	8.5F, 9.5F	Holmium:YAG laser	94.1% (32/34)	Outpatients	–	–
Park et al. [19]	66	7.9F–11.5F	Intact or lithoclast	86.4% (57/66)	–	–	–
Pearle et al. [54]	48	6.9–8.5F	Alexandrite laser	94% (45/48)	–	–	–
MacDermott et al. [55]	76	7.2F	Pulsed-dye laser	91% (69/76)	–	–	–
Bierkens et al. [56]	80	7.2F	Pulsed-dye laser	99% (79/80)	3.2	0% (0/80)	7% (6/80)
Biyani et al. [57]	25	6F	Holmium:YAG laser	100% (25/25)	–	–	–
Pardalidis et al. [18]	228[a] (238)	11.5F	USL, EHL	92% (219/238)	1.3	2.5% (6/238)	4.2% (10/238)
Peschel et al. [40]	40	6.5F, 9.5F	Intact, lithoclast	100% (40/40)	–	0% (0/40)	0% (0/40)
Turk and Jenkins [39]	96	7.5–9.5F	Intact, pulsed-dye laser	95% (93/96)	–	5.2% (5/96)	3.1% (3/96)
Pearle et al. [41]	32	6.9F, 11.5F	Intact, Alexandrite or Holmium: YAG laser, EHL	100% (29/29)	75% outpatients	25% (8/32)	0% (0/32)
Total	2879	–		95% (2740/2892)	–	6.1% (134/2205)	6.3% (144/2300)

[a] Includes three patients in whom the stone was treated from a percutaneous antegrade approach.
USL, ultrasonic lithotripsy; EHL, electrohydraulic lithotripsy.

In most ureteroscopy series, a ureteral stent is placed for at least a few days postprocedure. However, recent reports by Hosking et al. [23] and Wollin and Denstedt [24] suggest that placement of a ureteral stent may be unnecessary for uncomplicated ureteroscopic procedures. Among 93 patients undergoing uncomplicated ureteroscopy for distal ureteral stones, only 5% of patients required emergency-room visits, 6% of patients required hospitalization, and no patient required nephrostomy tube or stent placement as a result of obstruction postoperatively [23]. Although 57% of patients experienced discomfort postoperatively, 85% of patients in this subgroup were well controlled with oral narcotics.

Wollin and Denstedt [24] also showed that there was no advantage in the placement of a ureteral stent in 39 patients undergoing uncomplicated ureteroscopy who were randomized to stent or no stent. At 1-week follow-up, the stented group reported more flank and bladder symptoms than the unstented group, although at subsequent visits no difference in symptoms was detected between the two groups. In both groups, all patients were rendered free of stone, although one patient in each group required an emergency-room visit and/or hospitalization; one patient in the unstented group experienced persistent vomiting postoperatively, and one patient in the stented group developed urosepsis.

Shock Wave Lithotripsy

Reported success rates for SWL of distal ureteral calculi using a first-generation Dornier HM3 range from 77% to 100% (Table 2). The average re-treatment rate in these combined series was 10% and the auxiliary procedure rate was 6%. Complications occurring with SWL treatment are few, and consist primarily of postoperative renal colic and fever.

Although the majority of patients in these series were treated with a ureteral catheter in place, equally high success rates have been achieved with in situ SWL treatment [25, 26]. Marberger et al. [26] prospectively treated 161 patients with distal ureteral calculi (including patients with impacted stones and those with infection treated with nephrostomy drainage and antibiotics) by in situ SWL on a Siemens Lithostar (Siemens Medical Engineering Group, Erlangen, Germany) and reported a 3-month stone-free rate of 95%. Indeed, clinical practice guidelines do not support the routine use of ureteral stents with the intention of improving stone-free rates with SWL for ureteral stones [27].

Success rates for SWL using second- and third-generation lithotripters are slightly, but consistently, lower than those achieved with the Dornier HM3: 85.7% vs. 88.5% (Tables 2 and 3). Re-treatment rates average 16.5% and mean auxiliary procedure rates are 11.1%. Although no prospective randomized trials have compared first-generation lithotripters with newer-generation machines, Anderson et al. [25] noted stone-free rates of 96% for patients with distal ureteral stones treated on a Dornier HM3 versus 84% for patients treated on a Siemens Lithostar.

TABLE 2. Results of shock wave lithotripsy for distal ureteral calculi using a Dornier HM3 lithotripter

Author	Patients	Stone-free	Re-treatment rate	Auxiliary procedure	Ureteral catheter	Length of stay (days)	Complications
Miller and Hautmann [58]	119	84% (100/119)	12% (14/119)	6% (7/119)	0%	2.4	0% (0/119)
Manzone and Chiang [59]	131	77% (100/131)	–	–	69%	–	–
Pettersson and Tiselius [60]	28	100% (28/28)	4% (1/28)	14% (4/28)	79%	–	–
Becht et al. [9]	39	95% (37/39)	18% (7/39)	0% (0/30)	0%	–	–
El-Faqih et al. [38]	53	84% (37/44)	9% (5/53)	4% (2/53)	19%	1.2	–
Selli and Carini [61]	70	94% (66/70)	13% (9/70)	–	99%	–	–
Keeler et al. [62]	119	89% (106/119)	4.2% (5/119)	8.5% (10/119)	45%	–	1% (1/119)
Kapoor et al. [36]	20	90% (18/20)	25% (5/20)	10% (2/20)	40%	2.8	25% (5/20)
Landau et al. [63]	155	97% (150/155)	6% (10/155)	2% (3/155)	22%	1.3	1% (2/155)
Erturk et al. [64]	312	81% (199/245)	4% (14/312)	–	79%	–	5% (16/312)
Tiselius [65]	212	96.7% (205/212)	23% (49/212)	7% (15/212)	62%	–	–
Anderson et al. [25]	27	96% (26/27)	3% (2/65)	6% (4/65)	0%	–	0% (0/27)
Turk and Jenkins [39]	44	78%	–	–	–	–	–
Pearle et al. [41]	32	100% (29/29)	0% (0/29)	0% (0/29)	16%	–	–
Total	1361	88.5% (1135/1282)	9.9% (121/1221)	5.7% (47/830)	–	–	3.2% (24/752)

TABLE 3. Results of shock wave lithotripsy for distal ureteral calculi using second- or third-generation lithotripters

Author	Lithotripter	Patients	Stone-free	Re-treatment rate	Auxiliary procedure	Ureteral catheter	Length of stay (days)	Complications
Holden and Rao [66]	Lithostar	38	100% (38/38)	–	18% (7/38)	0%	–	–
Simon et al. [67]	Lithostar	141	83% (117/141)	14% (20/141)	7.1% (10/141)	5.7%	–	–
Netto et al. [37]	Lithostar	25	88% (22/25)	8% (2/25)	–	–	–	4.7% (6/129)
Mobley et al. [68]	Lithostar	6638	83% (4084/4921)	10%	9%	12.5%	–	–
Chang et al. [34]	Lithostar	32	59% (19/32)	0% (0/32)	41% (13/42)	0%	3	–
Farsi et al. [69]	Lithostar	101	80% (81/101)	–	–	–	–	–
Anderson et al. [25]	Lithostar	22	84% (18/22)	14% (3/22)	14% (3/22)	18%	Outpatients	0% (0/27)
Mogensen and Andersen [70]	Lithostar	77	82% (63/77)	1.2 tx/pt	21% (16/77)	10.4%	–	–
Bierkens et al. [56]	Lithostar	44	81% (36/44)	50% (22/44)	5% (2/44)	0%	Outpatients	–
Pardalidis et al. [18]	Lithostar	395	93% (368/395) 1 tx. 99% (391/395) 2 tx	6% (23/368)	1% (4/368)	–	Outpatients	4.3% (17/395)
Basar et al. [71]	Tripter XI	28	82% (23/28)	21% (6/28)	7% (2/28)	0%	–	0% (0/28)
Delivellotis et al. [17]	HM4	50	98% (49/50)	6% (3/50)	2% (1/50)	0%	Outpatients	0% (0/50)
Thomas et al. [72]	Medstone	130	85% (102/120)	3% (4/130)	10% (13/130)	32%	–	–
Eden et al. [20]	Modulith	313	74.8% single stones, 50% multiple stones	–	25.9% (81/313)	16%	Outpatients	4.4% (14/313)
Voce et al. [73]	MPL9000	285	97% (276/285)	34% (95/285)	3% (9/285)	4%	Outpatients	0% (0/285)
Frabboni et al. [74]	MPL9000	285	97% (276/285)	17% (49/285)	4% (12/285)	4%	Outpatients	0% (0/285)
Park et al. [19]	MPL9000	131	91.6% (120/131)	11.4% (15/131)	–	–	–	–
Turk and Jenkins [39]	HM3/MFL5000	91	73%	15% (14/91)	6.5% (6/91)	–	–	0% (0/91)
Peschel et al. [40]	MFL5000	40	90% (36/40)	0% (0/40)	10% (4/40)	–	–	0% (0/40)
Gnanapragasam et al. [75]	MFL5000	62 (67)	85.5% (53/62)	–	14.5% (9/62)	8%	Outpatients	0% (0/62)
Total	–	8908	85.7% (6238/7283)	16.5% (256/1552)	11.1% (192/1736)	–	–	2.2% (37/1705)

tx, treatment; pt, patients.

Open Ureterolithotomy

Ureterolithotomy is a salvage procedure reserved for the rare endourological and SWL failure. Several groups have reviewed their open-surgery experience in the era of endourology and SWL. Soon after the introduction of SWL, Assimos et al. [28] reviewed their surgical procedures for stones and found that ureterolithotomy comprised 2.6% of the 893 procedures for stones at their institution. Kane et al. [29] also performed eight ureterolithotomies, comprising 3% of their 799 surgical stone procedures between 1990 and 1993. The indications for ureterolithotomy included failed URS (two patients), failed URS and SWL (one patient), impacted stones (two patients), simultaneous anatrophic nephrolithotomy (two patients), and simultaneous prostatectomy (one patient). Likewise, Resnick and co-workers [30] performed seven ureterolithotomies between 1991 and 1995 for distal ureteral calculi. All stones were more than 2 cm in diameter, and the indications for open surgery included a failed endoscopic approach (five patients), associated ureteral stricture (one patient), and concurrent colon surgery (one patient). With currently available technology, ureterolithotomy for distal ureteral calculi should be exceedingly rare, comprising less than 1% of cases.

Laparoscopic Ureterolithotomy

Laparoscopic ureterolithotomy has been described anecdotally as an alternative to open ureterolithotomy for endourological failures [31–33]. While the majority of reported cases have involved proximal ureteral stones, laparoscopic techniques have also been successfully applied to distal ureteral stones. Indeed, the distal ureter is quite commonly visualized during laparoscopic pelvic lymph node dissection and other laparoscopic pelvic procedures. Laparoscopic ureterolithotomy has been performed via both a transperitoneal and a retroperitoneal approach [31, 32]. Typically, a ureteral stent is placed alongside the stone preoperatively, and the ureterotomy is left open, or is closed over a stent after stone removal, and a drain is left in place.

Treatment Selection

Ureteroscopy vs. SWL: Review of Retrospective Series

A number of investigators have retrospectively compared their single institution's experience with SWL and URS for distal ureteral stones [18–20, 25, 34–39]. Several series demonstrated comparable stone-free rates for URS and SWL [25, 36, 38]. Using a Dornier HM3, three series demonstrated stone-free rates between 90% and 97%, with a 0% to 7% re-treatment rate for SWL versus a 95% to 100% stone-free rate and a 0% to 6% re-treatment rate for URS.

Other series demonstrated superior stone-free rates for URS over SWL [34, 35, 39]. Turk and Jenkins [39] concluded that URS was more efficacious than SWL for the treatment of distal ureteral calculi based on their recent series of 187 patients with distal ureteral calculi treated with SWL (44 on a Dornier HM3 and 47 on a Dornier MFL5000) or URS (n = 96). Although stone-free rates favored URS (95%) over SWL (83% for the HM3, 77% for the MFL5000), complications occurred only in the URS group (5.2%), including four ureteral perforations and one stricture.

Some authors stratified their results by stone size or multiplicity and based treatment recommendations on the outcomes. Eden et al. [26] reviewed 447 patients with distal ureteral calculi treated with SWL on a Storz Modulith (Storz Medical, Krenzlingln, Switzerland) SL20 (n = 313) or with URS (n = 134). For single stones, stone-free rates of 75% and 90% were achieved for SWL and URS, respectively; for multiple stones, SWL resulted in a 50% stone-free rate versus an 89% stone-free rate with URS. Stone-free rates for SWL decreased with increasing stone size. For stones <8mm diameter, stone-free rates of 89% to 100% were achieved with SWL compared with 11% to 75% for stones >8mm diameter. Likewise, re-treatment rates increased from 11.5% for small stones to 54% for large stones. In contrast, URS outcomes were independent of size. Thus, the authors concluded that SWL should constitute first-line therapy for small (<8mm), single, distal ureteral calculi, while URS should be reserved for large or multiple stones.

Pardalidis et al. [18] also advocated selective therapy based on stone size. In their series of 633 distal ureteral calculi treated with URS (n = 228) or SWL on a Siemens Lithostar (n = 395), a 99% stone-free rate with a 6% re-treatment rate was achieved for SWL compared with a 92% single procedure stone-free rate for URS. Complications in the SWL group were mild, and consisted of renal colic or fever; in the URS group, ureteral perforation or stricture occurred in 1.7% and 0.8% of patients, respectively. For stones ≤10mm in size, stone-free rates were similar for the two modalities: 100% for SWL versus 97% for URS. However, for stones >10mm, URS was slightly more efficacious than SWL (stone-free rates of 91% versus 85%, respectively). Consequently, the authors recommended SWL for stones ≤10mm and URS for stones >10mm.

Park et al. [19] also favored SWL for small stones, reserving URS for large stones or SWL failures. In their 2-year experience treating ureteral stones with SWL on a Dornier MPL9000 (n = 131 distal ureteral stones) or URS (n = 66 distal ureteral stones), a stone-free rate for distal ureteral calculi of 92% was achieved for SWL versus 86% for URS. Re-treatment rates were comparable for the two treatment groups: 11% for SWL and 12% for URS. A stone-free rate of 94% was achieved with SWL for stones <1 cm, but this dropped to 56% for stones >1 cm. Combined URS stone-free rates for ureteral stones in all locations were unaffected by stone size, but no stratified data were presented for distal ureteral stones. Complications in the series included steinstrasse in 2.3% of SWL patients and ureteral perforation, stricture, or sepsis in 7% of URS patients.

URS vs. SWL: Review of Prospective Series

Only three prospective series have directly compared the efficacies of SWL and URS for the treatment of distal ureteral calculi. Deliveliotis et al. [17] carried out a prospective, nonrandomized trial of 100 patients with distal ureteral calculi treated consecutively, first with URS and later with SWL on a Dornier HM4 lithotripter. Single-procedure stone-free rates of 100% for URS and 92% for SWL were achieved, but with the addition of a single SWL treatment in six cases, a total stone-free rate of 98% was achieved in the SWL group. Procedural time, complication rate, and convalescence time favored SWL over URS. No complications occurred in the SWL group, while two URS patients (4%) sustained a ureteral perforation. The authors concluded that SWL, using an HM4 lithotripter, should constitute first-line therapy for distal ureteral calculi.

Peschel et al. [40] recently conducted a prospective, randomized trial comparing SWL on a Dornier MFL5000 ($n = 40$) with URS ($n = 40$) for distal ureteral stones. Patients in each group were further randomized by stone size into groups with stones <5 mm and stones >5 mm ($n = 20$ in each group). Overall stone-free rates were 100% for URS and 90% for SWL: 85% of SWL patients with small stones versus 95% of patients with large stones were rendered stone-free. Mean procedural time favored URS in both size categories, and no complications occurred in any group. Patient satisfaction reflected treatment success: 100% of URS and 85% of SWL patients were satisfied with their procedure. The authors favored URS as first-line treatment for distal ureteral stones based on higher stoner-free rates, shorter time to become stone-free, and greater patient satisfaction.

Pearle et al. [41] also performed a prospective, randomized trial comparing the two treatment modalities for distal ureteral stones. Of note, SWL was performed on an unmodified HM3 lithotripter using a modified Stryker frame. A total of 64 patients with stones ≤15 mm diameter were randomized to SWL ($n = 32$) or URS ($n = 32$). Single procedure stone-free rates of 100% were achieved for 27 patients in each group who had adequate follow-up. Only five SWL and four URS patients had a ureteral stent in place at the time of treatment. Operative time was statistically significantly shorter for SWL compared with URS (by 30 min). In addition, SWL patients experienced less flank pain and dysuria, had fewer complications, recovered more quickly, and were more satisfied with their procedure than URS patients, although the differences did not reach statistical significance. Despite comparable stone-free rates, the authors favored HM3 SWL over URS for stones ≤15 mm diameter based on more favorable secondary outcomes for SWL.

In all series performing cost analyses, SWL was more costly than URS by $1000–$2000 [34–36, 42, 43]. However, taking into consideration the need for stent removal in most URS patients and the higher incidence of overnight hospitalization, the cost differential is lessened although not eliminated.

Established Guidelines

In 1997, the American Urological Association (AUA) convened the Ureteral Stones Clinical Guidelines Panel to formulate guidelines regarding the management of distal ureteral stones based on the therapeutic options reported in the literature [27]. Abstractable data were derived from 327 articles published between 1966 and 1993.

For distal ureteral calculi, the panel concluded that patients in whom active treatment is indicated should undergo SWL or ureteroscopy as first-line therapy. Blind extraction procedures (blind-basketing) were not considered acceptable forms of treatment for distal ureteral stones, and open surgery was recommended only as a salvage procedure or in unusual circumstances. No specific recommendations regarding the choice of URS versus SWL were made for stones <1 cm. However, because of the higher re-treatment rate associated with SWL therapy of stones >1 cm, the panel suggested that URS may be preferable to SWL for some stones in this size group.

Recommendations

In summary, the published literature supports both URS and SWL as first-line therapy for distal ureteral calculi that fail to pass spontaneously. However, for single stones ≤15 mm diameter, comparable efficacy and reduced patient morbidity make in situ HM3 SWL the preferred treatment for this subgroup of patients, despite a modest cost differential favoring URS. If only newer-generation lithotripters are available, the advantage of SWL over URS is less well documented. For multiple stones, or stones >15 mm diameter, URS is the preferred first-line treatment. In the rare event that SWL and URS fail, laparoscopic ureterolithotomy provides salvage therapy in most cases. At this time, open ureterolithotomy should be reserved only for endoscopic and laparoscopic failures.

Conclusions

The optimal therapy for distal ureteral calculi is controversial; both URS and SWL are associated with high success rates and low complication rates. However, for single stones ≤15 mm diameter, HM3 SWL offers comparable efficacy to URS but with less patient morbidity. Whether newer-generation lithotripters offer comparable efficacy and efficiency to the HM3, and confer the same advantage over URS, is debatable; only a direct comparison between the HM3 and newer lithotripters will definitively answer that question. Although cost continues to favor URS, the differences are likely to lessen as the capital cost of lithotripters decreases. For stones >15 mm or multiple stones, URS provides optimal first-line treatment. Open or laparoscopic ureterolithotomy is reserved as salvage therapy for endoscopic and SWL failures.

References

1. Murphy LJT (1972) The history of urology. Charles C. Thomas. Springfield
2. Perez-Castro Ellendt E, Martinez-Pineiro JA (1980) Transurethral ureteroscopy. A current urological procedure. Arch Esp Urol 33:445–460

3. Keating MA, Heney NM, Young HH II, Kerr WS Jr, O'Leary MP, Dretler SP (1986) Ureteroscopy: the initial experience. J Urol 135:689–693
4. Blute ML, Segura JW, Patterson DE (1988) Ureteroscopy. J Urol 139:510–512
5. Daniels GF Jr, Garnett JE, Carter MF (1988) Ureteroscopic results and complications: experience with 130 cases. J Urol 139:710–713
6. Lingeman JE, Sonda LP, Kahnoski RJ, Coury TA, Newman DM, Mosbaugh PG, Mertz JH, Steele RE, Frank B (1986) Ureteral stone management: emerging concepts. J Urol 135:1172–1174
7. Politis G, Griffith DP (1987) Ureteroscopy in management of ureteral calculi. Urology 30:39–42
8. Miller K, Bubeck JR, Hautmann R (1986) Extracorporeal shockwave lithotripsy of distal ureteral calculi. Eur Urol 12:305–307
9. Becht E, Moll V, Neisius D, Ziegler M (1988) Treatment of prevesical ureteral calculi by extracorporeal shock wave lithotripsy. J Urol 139:916–918
10. Jenkins AD, Gillenwater JY (1988) Extracorporeal shock wave lithotripsy in the prone position: treatment of stones in the distal ureter or anomalous kidney. J Urol 139:911–915
11. Leveillee RJ, Zabbo A, Barrette D (1994) Stryker frame adaptation of the HM3 lithotriptor for treatment of distal ureteral calculi. J Urol 151:391–393
12. Pearle MS, McClennan BL, Roehrborn CG, Clayman RV (1997) Bolus injection v. drip infusion contrast administration for ureteral stone targeting during shockwave lithotripsy. J Endourol 11:163–166
13. Swanson SK (1992) Excretory urography during extracorporeal shock-wave lithotripsy: a localization alternative. Urology 39:185–186
14. Morse RM, Resnick MI (1991) Ureteral calculi: natural history and treatment in an era of advanced technology. J Urol 145:263–265
15. Miller OF, Kane CJ (1999) Time to stone passage for observed ureteral calculi: a guide for patient education. J Urol 162:688–690
16. Leventhal EK, Rozanski TA, Crain TW, Deshon GE Jr (1995) Indwelling ureteral stents as definitive therapy for distal ureteral calculi. J Urol 153:34–36
17. Deliveliotis C, Stavropoulos NI, Koutsokalis G, Kostakopoulos A, Dimopoulos C (1996) Distal ureteral calculi: ureteroscopy vs. ESWL. A prospective analysis. Int Urol Nephrol 28:627–631
18. Pardalidis NP, Kosmaoglou EV, Kapotis CG (1999) Endoscopy vs. extracorporeal shockwave lithotripsy in the treatment of distal ureteral stones: ten years' experience. J Endourol 13:161–164
19. Park H, Park M, Park T (1998) Two-year experience with ureteral stones: extracorporeal shockwave lithotripsy v. ureteroscopic manipulation. J Endourol 12:501–504
20. Eden CG, Mark IR, Gupta RR, Eastman J, Shrotri NC, Tiptaft RC (1998) Intracorporeal or extracorporeal lithotripsy for distal ureteral calculi? Effect of stone size and multiplicity on success rates. J Endourol 12:307–312
21. Netto NR, Claro J, de Almeida Claro, Esteves SC, Andrade EFM (1997) Ureteroscopic stone removal in the distal ureter. Why change? J Urol 157:2081–2083
22. Jung P, Wolff JM, Mattelaer P, Jakse G (1996) Role of lasertripsy in the management of ureteral calculi: experience with Alexandrite laser system in 232 patients. J Endourol 10:345–348
23. Hosking DH, McColm SE, Smith WE (1999) Is stenting following ureteroscopy for removal of distal ureteral calculi necessary? J Urol 161:48–50

24. Wollin T, Denstedt JD (1999) A prospective randomized controlled trial comparing stented versus non-stented ureteroscopic lithotripsy. J Endourol 13(Suppl 1):A41

25. Anderson KR, Keetch DW, Albala DM, Chandhoke PS, McClennan BL, Clayman RV (1994) Optimal therapy for the distal ureteral stone: extracorporeal shock wave lithotripsy versus ureteroscopy. J Urol 152:62–65

26. Marberger M, Hofbauer J, Turck CH, Albrecht W (1992) Minimally invasive therapy 1:159–167

27. Segura JW, Preminger GM, Assimos DG, Dretler SP, Kahn RI, Lingeman JE, Macaluso JN Jr (1997) Ureteral Stones Clinical Guidelines Panel summary report on the management of ureteral calculi. American Urological Association. J Urol 158:1915–1921

28. Assimos DG, Boyce WH, Harrison LH, McCullough DL, Kroovand RL, Sweat KR (1989) The role of open stone surgery since extracorporeal shock wave lithotripsy. J Urol 142:263–267

29. Kane CJ, Bolton DM, Stoller ML (1995) Current indications for open stone surgery in an endourology center. Urology 45:218–221

30. Paik ML, Wainstein MA, Spirnak JP, Hampel N, Resnick MI (1998) Current indications for open stone surgery in the treatment of renal and ureteral calculi. J Urol 159:374–378

31. Raboy A, Ferzli GS, Ioffreda R, Albert PS (1992) Laparoscopic ureterolithotomy. Urology 39:223–225

32. Gaur DD (1993) Retroperitoneal endoscopic ureterolithotomy: our experience in 12 patients. J Endourol 7:501–503

33. Bellman GC, Smith AD (1994) Special considerations in the technique of laparoscopic ureterolithotomy. J Urol 151:146–149

34. Chang SC, Ho CM, Kuo HC (1993) Ureteroscopic treatment of lower ureteral calculi in the era of extracorporeal shock wave lithotripsy: from a developing country's point of view. J Urol 150:1395–1398

35. Francesca F, Grasso M, Lucchelli M, Broglia L, Cammelli L, Zoppei G, Rigatti P (1993) Cost–efficacy comparison of extracorporeal shock wave lithotripsy and endoscopic laser lithotripsy in distal ureteral stones. J Endourol 7:289–291

36. Kapoor DA, Leech JE, Yap WT, Rose JF, Kabler R, Mowad JJ (1992) Cost and efficacy of extracorporeal shock wave lithotripsy versus ureteroscopy in the treatment of lower ureteral calculi. J Urol 148:1095–1096

37. Netto NR Jr, Claro JF, Lemos GC, Cortado PL (1991) Treatment options for ureteral calculi: endourology or extracorporeal shock wave lithotripsy. J Urol 146:5–7

38. El-Faqih SR, Husain I, Ekman PE, Sharma ND, Chakrabarty A, Talic R (1988) Primary choice of intervention for distal ureteric stone: ureteroscopy or ESWL? Br J Urol 62:13–18

39. Turk TM, Jenkins AD (1999) A comparison of ureteroscopy to in situ extracorporeal shock wave lithotripsy for the treatment of distal ureteral calculi. J Urol 161:45–46

40. Peschel R, Janetschek G, Bartsch G (1999) Extracorporeal shock wave lithotripsy versus ureteroscopy for distal ureteral calculi: a prospective randomized study. J Urol 162:1909–1912

41. Pearle MS, Nadler R, Bercowsky E, Chen C, Dunn M, Figmshau RS, Hoenig DM, McDougall EM, Mutz J, Nakada SY, Shalhav AL, Sundaram C, Wolf JS Jr, Clayman RV (2001) Prospective, randomized, trial comparing shockwave lithotripsy with a Dornier HM3 and ureteroscopy for the management of distal ureteral calculi. J Urol (in press)

42. Nesbit J, Drago JR (1989) Treatment options for ureteral calculi: endourology or extracorporeal shock wave lithotripsy. J Endourol 3:47–50
43. Wolf JS Jr, Carroll PR, Stoller ML (1995) Cost-effectiveness v. patient preference in the choice of treatment for distal ureteral calculi: a literature-based decision analysis. J Endourol 9:243–248
44. Dretler SP (1990) An evaluation of ureteral laser lithotripsy: 225 consecutive patients. J Urol 143:267–272
45. Dretler SP, Bhatta KM (1991) Clinical experience with high-power (140mJ), large-fiber (320 micron) pulsed-dye laser lithotripsy. J Urol 146:1228–1231
46. Fugelso P, Neal PM (1991) Endoscopic laser lithotripsy: safe, effective therapy for ureteral calculi. J Urol 145:949–951
47. Garvin TJ, Clayman RV (1991) Balloon dilation of the distal ureter to 24F: an effective method for ureteroscopic stone retrieval. J Urol 146:742–745
48. Esuvaranathan K, Tan EC, Tan PK, Tung KH (1992) Does transurethral laser ureterolithotripsy justify its cost? J Urol 148:1091–1094
49. Benizri E, Wodey J, Amiel J, Toubol J (1993) Comparison of 2 pulsed lasers for lithotripsy of ureteral calculi: report on 154 patients. J Urol 150:1803–1805
50. Yiu MK, Liu PL, Yiu TF, Chan AY (1996) Clinical experience with holmium:YAG laser lithotripsy of ureteral calculi. Lasers Surg Med 19:103–106
51. Harmon WJ, Sershon PD, Blute ML, Patterson DE, Segura JW (1997) Ureteroscopy: current practice and long-term complications. J Urol 157:28–32
52. Kupeli B, Biri H, Isen K, Onaran M, Alkibay T, Karaoglan U, Bozkirli I (1998) Treatment of ureteral stones: comparison of extracorporeal shock wave lithotripsy and endourologic alternatives. Eur Urol 34:474–479
53. Yip KH, Lee CW, Tam PC (1998) Holmium laser lithotripsy for ureteral calculi: an outpatient procedure. J Endourol 12:241–246
54. Pearle MS, Sech SM, Cobb CG, Riley JR, Clark PJ, Preminger GM, Drach GW, Roehrborn CG (1998) Safety and efficacy of the Alexandrite laser for the treatment of renal and ureteral calculi. Urology 51:33–38
55. MacDermott JP, Grove J, Clark PB (1993) Laser lithotripsy with the Candela MDL-2000 lasertripter. Br J Urol 71:512–515
56. Bierkens AF, Hendrikx AJ, De La Rosette JJ, Stultiens GN, Beerlage HP, Arends AJ, Debruyne FM (1998) Treatment of mid- and lower ureteric calculi: extracorporeal shock-wave lithotripsy vs. laser ureteroscopy. A comparison of costs, morbidity and effectiveness. Br J Urol 81:31–35
57. Biyani CS, Cornford PA, Powell CS (1998) Ureteroscopic holmium lasertripsy for ureteric stones. Initial experience. Scand J Urol Nephrol 32:92–93
58. Miller K, Hautmann R (1987) Treatment of distal ureteral calculi with ESWL: experience with more than consecutive cases. World J Urol 5:259–261
59. Manzone JJ, Chiang B (1988) Extracorporeal shock wave lithotripsy of stones in the upper, mid- and lower ureter. J Endourol 2:107–111
60. Pettersson B, Tiselius HG (1988) Extracorporeal shock wave lithotripsy of proximal and distal ureteral stones. Eur Urol 14:184–188
61. Selli C, Carini M (1988) Treatment of lower ureteral calculi with extracorporeal shock wave lithotripsy. J Urol 140:280–282
62. Keeler LL, McNamara TC, Dorey FO, Milsten RE (1990) De novo extracorporeal shock wave lithotripsy for lower ureteral calculi: treatment of choice. J Endourol 4:71–77

63. Landau EH, Pode D, Lencovsky Z, Katz G, Meretyk S, Shapiro A (1992) Extracorporeal shock-wave lithotripsy (ESWL) monotherapy for stones in lower ureter. Urology 40:132–136
64. Erturk E, Herrman E, Cockett AT (1993) Extracorporeal shock wave lithotripsy for distal ureteral stones. J Urol 149:1425–1426
65. Tiselius HG (1993) Anesthesia-free extracorporeal shock wave lithotripsy of distal ureteral stones without a ureteral catheter. J Endourol 7:285–287
66. Holden D, Rao PN (1989) Ureteral stones: the results of primary in situ extracorporeal shock wave lithotripsy. J Urol 142:37–39
67. Simon J, Vanden Bossche M, Schulman CC (1990) Shockwave treatment of ureteric stones in situ with second-generation lithotriptor. Eur Urol 17:200–202
68. Mobley TB, Myers DA, Grine WB, Jenkins JM, Jordan WR (1993) Low-energy lithotripsy with the Lithostar: treatment results with 19962 renal and ureteral calculi. J Urol 149:1419–1424
69. Farsi HM, Mosli HA, Alzimaity M, Bahnassay AA, Ibrahim MA (1994) In situ extracorporeal shock wave lithotripsy for primary ureteric calculi. Urology 43:776–781
70. Mogensen P, Andersen JT (1994) Primary in situ extracorporeal shock wave lithotripsy for ureteral calculi. Scand J Urol Nephrol Suppl 157:159–163
71. Basar I, Gurpinar T, Erkan A (1992) In situ prone ESWL for the treatment of lower ureteral stones: experience with 28 patients. Int Urol Nephrol 24:369–373
72. Thomas R, Macaluso JN, Vandenberg T, Salvatore FT (1993) An innovative approach to management of lower third ureteral calculi. J Urol 149:1427–1430
73. Voce S, Dal Pozzo C, Arnone S, Montanari F (1993) "In situ" echo-guided extracorporeal shock wave lithotripsy of ureteral stones. Methods and results with Dornier MPL 9000. Scand J Urol Nephrol 27:469–473
74. Frabboni R, Santi V, Ronchi M, Gaiani S, Costanza N, Ferrari G, Ferrari P, Corrado G, Concetti S, Fornarola V (1994) In situ echo-guided extracorporeal shock wave lithotripsy of ureteric stones with the Dornier MPL 9000: a multicentric study group. Br J Urol 73:487–493
75. Gnanapragasam VJ, Ramsden PD, Murthy LS, Thomas DJ (1999) Primary in situ extracorporeal shock wave lithotripsy in the management of ureteric calculi: results with a third-generation lithotripter. BJU Int 84:770–774

Percutaneous Nephrolithotripsy (PNL): What Factors Make PNL Difficult and What Are the Ways to Prevent and Solve Those Problems?

Akito Yamaguchi[1], Kaoru Miyazaki[1], Hiroyuki Meiri[2], Jiro Uozumi[2], and Zenjiro Masaki[2]

Summary. There are two factors that make percutaneous nephrolithotripsy (PNL) difficult. One is an inevitable difficulty in cases where the percutaneous approach to the kidney is limited by an anatomical hazard such as a kidney which is located higher than normal, or a visceral organ which lies on the line of the planned nephrostomy tract. The other is a difficulty which has been secondarily brought about in essentially easy cases by neglect of the basic technical rules for PNL. In a general urology department, the latter is far more frequent than the former, and because of this, general urologists may have the wrong view that PNL is difficult.

The reasons why basic techniques have to be followed, especially in creating a nephrostomy tract, are described. One of the difficult conditions caused by neglect of the rules is the case where the guide wire, after having entered the collecting system, is then forced outside the system and the tract is dilated. This is particularly liable to occur when the guide wire gets into the peripelvic space. Ways to prevent and deal with this problem are described.

PNL is an established method for the treatment of renal staghorn calculi, and we believe that it is not essentially a difficult procedure to perform as long as the basic technical rules are followed.

Key Words. Percutaneous nephrolithotomy (nephrolithotripsy), Staghorn calculi, Nephrostomy, Basic technique, Complication

[1] Department of Urology, Harasanshin Hospital, 1-8 Taihaku-cho, Hakata-ku, Fukuoka 812-0033, Japan
[2] Department of Urology, Saga Medical School, 5-1-1 Nabeshima, Saga 849-8501, Japan

Introduction

Percutaneous nephrolithotripsy (PNL) is currently the established method for the treatment of renal staghorn calculi, although technological advances continue to appear. During the years before extracorporeal shockwave lithotripsy (ESWL) became widely available, most urolithiasis was treated with PNL regardless of stone size, anatomical variation in the urinary tract, and other conditions that influence treatment selection. The advent of ESWL dramatically changed the mode of stone therapy, and the use of PNL for the treatment of urolithiasis decreased considerably. Since then, ESWL has occupied the main position in stone treatment even for the treatment of staghorn calculi, and as a result, general urologists have rarely had the chance to obtain experience of PNL.

Recently, however, the use of PNL is increasing, especially for treatment of staghorn calculi. This tendency may be because PNL has been reevaluated, and is now seen as a more efficient treatment modality for staghorn calculi [1], either as a single procedure or as a combined method with ESWL (Fig. 1).

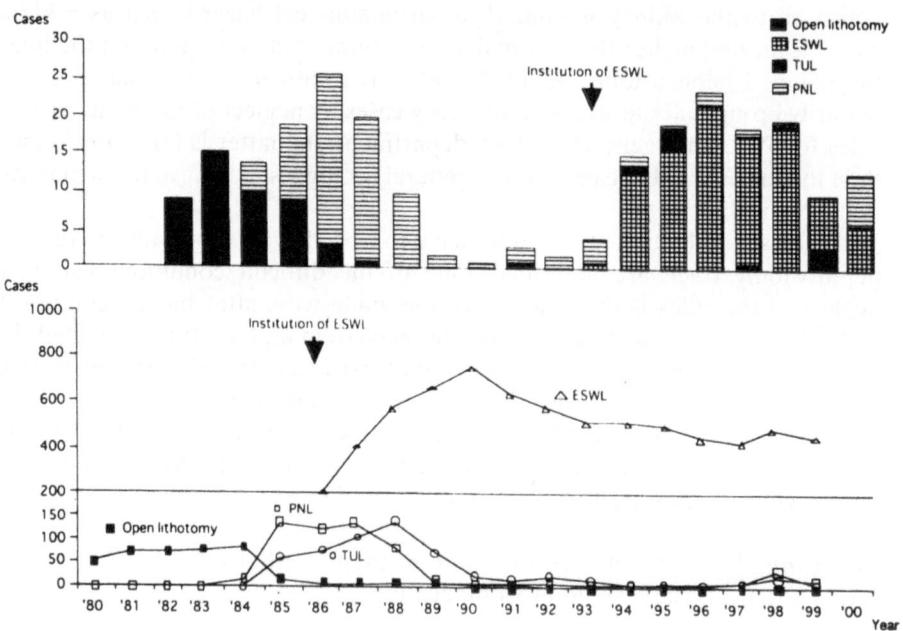

Fig. 1. Historical changes in the treatment of urolithiasis. The *upper* bar graph shows the yearly change in the number of cases with renal stones (ureteral stones excluded) treated by various modalities in the Saga Medical School, where the introduction of extracorporeal shockwave lithotripsy (ESWL) was relatively late. The *lower* line graph is the yearly change in the number of cases of all urinary tract stones, treated by different methods, in the Harasanshin Hospital, where ESWL was introduced immediately after it became available. *TUL*, transurethral ureterolithotripsy; *PNL*, percutaneous nephrolithotripsy

This tendency has also influenced decision-making in selecting the mode of stone treatment, and PNL has now regained its position as the main treatment modality for staghorn calculi [2]. Because of its historical background, PNL is now a method which must be learned by those who have little experience of PNL and who favor ESWL.

In this situation, it may be important to review what factors make PNL difficult, because the preference of young doctors for ESWL is often because of a misunderstanding that PNL requires special expertise.

There are two main factors which make PNL difficult. One is the neglect of the basic essential principles, and the other is the occasional truly difficult situation. For a better understanding of PNL, one should start by clearly distinguishing these two factors, although both of them can make the techniques difficult.

Neglect of Basic Techniques Makes PNL Difficult

The basic techniques to be followed in PNL are listed in Table 1. Since the success of PNL largely depends on how well the nephrostomy is made, the list is largely concerned with this subject. There are good reasons why all these basic techniques must be followed.

TABLE 1. Basic techniques essential for successful percutaneous nephrolithotripsy (PNL)

1. Preoperative assessment
    (1) The calyx to be punctured should be identified by ultrasonography in relation to the findings in IVP or RP (oblique position)
    (2) It should be confirmed by CT in the prone position that no visceral organ is interposed in the puncture line

2. Basic principles of an echo-guided puncture of the calyx
    (1) The puncture site is usually caudal to the 12th rib and on the posterior axilla line or a more dorsal aspect
    (2) The ideal puncture site is the posterior calyx cranial from the lowermost one
    (3) It is desirable that the renal pelvis is identifiable in the same echo-image depicting the target calyx
    (4) The depth of the puncture is up to the calyx, but not reaching the pelvis
    (5) The best timing for the needle puncture is at the end of an exhalation phase
    (6) When the first and second punctures are not successful, a repeat puncture should be done only after anatomically reconstructing the image of the puncture line[a]

3. Insertion of a guide wire and tract dilation
    (1) The guide wire should be advanced far enough in the pelvioureteral direction
    (2) The tract should be as straight as possible, and easily dilated without unusual resistance
    (3) A safety guide wire should be inserted before dilating the tract to more than 12F

4. Lithotripsy
    (1) Lithotripsy should only be carried out following rational planning
    (2) Irrigation should be under the minimum pressure necessary to stop venous bleeding

[a] A fluoroscopically guided puncture is described in the section "when initial access to the collecting system fails."
IVP, intravenous pyelography; RP, retrograde pyelography; CT, computed tomography.

Preoperative Assessment

It is essential for a successful procedure that the operator has a three-dimensional image of the collecting system. Ultrasonographic visualization of the calices may not be difficult, but confirming whether the correct calyx is being targeted is often difficult. Preoperative simulation of the puncture using all available information from intravenous pyelography (IVP), retrograde pyelography (RP), or computed tomography (CT) is mandatory. Identification of the posterior calices is facilitated by IVP or RP in an oblique position. In some cases a visceral organ is interposed in the nephrostomy tract. This is not a frequent occurrence, but should be checked by prone CT films to avoid rare complications such as splenic or colon injury.

Basic Principles of Echo-Guided Puncture

The reason why the puncture of the posterior calyx would be optimum is that it is usually located on a straight line between the puncture site and the renal pelvis (Fig. 2). Therefore, the pelvis is identifiable in the same plane as that on which the target calyx is focused. In addition, this tract passes through the safest zone, which corresponds to the area between the ventral and dorsal segment arterial supplies [3]. To approach the uretero-pelvic junction, it may be ideal to puncture the upper calyx, but the 12th rib often limits this procedure. This is the reason why the calyx next to the lowermost one is chosen. Puncture of the stone-bearing lower calyx is occasionally necessary, but the procedure is sometimes associated with difficult tract dilation (see below).

It is the general rule to expand the collecting system with an occlusion balloon indwelled in the ureter before the puncture. When the contrast medium is infused, care should be taken not to allow air into the perfusate. If this occurs, the air will collect in the targeted calyx, and will usually locate at the highest part

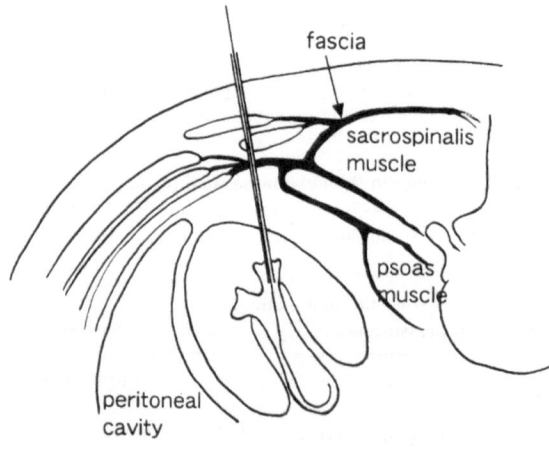

Fig. 2. The right nephrostomy tract. A tract through the posterior calyx reaches the renal pelvis in a straight line. If the dermal puncture site shifts too far medially, the tract has to pass through the tough fascial structures. If it shifts too far to the lateral side, the tract may injure visceral organs

of the collecting system when the patient is in a prone position. The air bubble will blur visualization of calyx with ultrasonography. In cases of puncture with the fluoroscopic guide, the target calyx tends to become lost from contrast visualization because the contrast medium, which has a high specific gravity, collects in the anterior calices. In such a case, the occlusion balloon should be advanced close to the target calyx to make it more opaque. Outlining the calyx with air [4] may be possible, but the result is not necessarily clear enough for practical use.

Puncture at a site caudal to the 12th rib can be done without fear of injuring the pleura. Puncture at a point which is more dorsal than the posteroaxillar line will avoid injury to the laterally positioned visceral organs. Too distant a shift to the dorsomedial side for the puncture site makes the approach to the pelvis difficult for two reasons. One is because the tract might possibly pass through the tough fascial structure of the sacrospinalis muscle, making dilation difficult (Fig. 2), and the other is because the lines from the dermal puncture site to the calyx and from the calyx to the renal pelvis may be at an angle.

Puncture of the collecting system should always be via a calyx in order to avoid direct puncture of the renal pelvis. The depth of the puncture must be limited to the caliceal level and not extend to the pelvis. This is a basic rule that is apt to be ignored even by experienced practitioners. Since many vascular structures are present around the renal pelvis and the infundibulum of the calyx [3], direct puncture of the renal pelvis without going through the calyx often results in injury to these vascular structures. However, a caliceal approach can avoid these complications.

The short interval of respiratory standstill at the end of an exhalation is the best time to make the puncture. The needle should be advanced rapidly, and as deep as the stopper attached to the needle allows. A slow maneuver might possibly push the kidney away, thus dislocating the target. A puncture at the moment of deepest inhalation needs special care that the upward movement of the kidney in the following exhalation phase does dislodge the needle tip that has already been inserted into the target calyx. Therefore, after a successful puncture in an inhalation phase, the guide wire should be inserted quickly before the next exhalation. Alternatively, the needle tip without the stylet can be further advanced by approximately 1 or 2 cm after a successful puncture, in preparation for the upward movement of the kidney at the next exhalation phase.

Confirmation that the needle tip is in the target calyx is obtained by a urine outflow from the needle. When a urine backflow is not observed, the needle, after the stylet has been pulled out, is withdrawn very slowly. Because 1 or 2 s are required for urine to pass through the thin needle, one should pause at every small back-movement of the needle. Sometime, it is possible to feel a faint reduction of resistance just when the needle tip moves into a hollow space, i.e., the collecting system. Feeling the needle tip contacting the stone suggests that the needle tip is within the collecting system even when urine does not flow back. Needle puncture can be repeated, again aiming at the target calyx, two or three times. However, if these repeat procedures fail, the puncture should be done differently, i.e., the direction or depth of the puncture should be changed after further consideration of the anatomy of the patient. If a needle with a beveled tip had been used, it should be exchanged to one with a diamond tip. A beveled tip often deviates from the ideal tract line owing to lateral forces created by its wedge shape.

Insertion of a Guide Wire and Tract Dilation

An indispensable condition for inserting a guide wire is that one should be able to advance it without any resistance, except when the stone itself blocks the passage of the guide wire. When resistance is felt at the tip of the guide wire, as if pushing against soft tissue, relocation of the needle tip or changing the direction of the needle is recommended. It should be remembered that perforation of the collecting system by a guide wire could be a factor that makes the subsequent PNL difficult. If an unsuitable tract is dilated over a guide wire that is improperly inserted, following procedures also become exceedingly difficult.

Ideally, a guide wire should be advanced into the ureter, but it is often the case that the wire goes into the upper calyx instead of directing to the ureter. Usually this does not cause any trouble, as long as the guide wire is not withdrawn during tract dilation. What is important is that the guide wire should be inserted long enough in the collecting system. In standard procedures, a guide wire with a flexible tip is generally used. However, various kinds of guide wire with different characteristics can be used in different situations. For instance, Radifocus (TERUMO, Japan) guide wire has a very smooth surface, giving less resistance upon insertion, but it tends to slip out of the collecting system. A stiffer guide wire may be easier to use for tract dilation.

When the punctured calyx is full of stones, and only a very narrow space is available between the stones and the mucosa of the calyx, the advancement of a guide wire is often blocked by a stone. Forcible pushing can deliver the guide wire outside the collecting system after piercing its wall. Therefore, while the guide wire is gently pushed against a stone, the direction of the needle is changed so that the wire slips along the surface of the stone. The best way is to advance the guide wire along the dorsal surface of the stone. When the guide wire is obviously blocked despite several attempts, one can let the wire coil itself inside the target calyx. The way of dealing with this situation is described below.

During dilation, the tract should be kept straight by fluoroscopic visualization. If this principle is followed, dilation of the tract usually straightforward. Any difficulty in dilating the tract could be a sign of trouble, except when the fascia on the tract is not satisfactorily incised. The most frequent reason for this difficulty is bending of the tract (Fig. 3). The tract should be straight in all three dimensions, and the patient's respiration should be adjusted to straighten it. Since the tract could easily be dilated up to 12 F, a safety guide wire should be inserted at this time. Any dilation larger than 12 F has to be done very slowly, with a pause at each stepwise enlargement.

FIG. 3. A bent nephrostomy tract. The tract should be kept straight during dilation to avoid a case like the one shown here

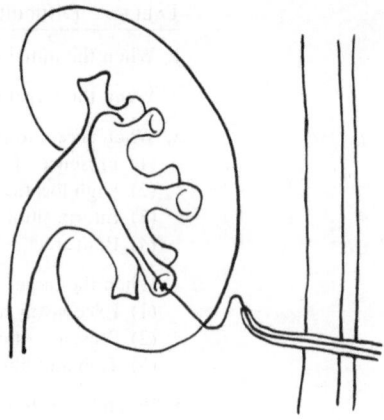

Lithotripsy

Nowadays, PNL is usually indicated for large stones. Thus, the extraction of stones as well as their disintegration are laborious tasks. Therefore, an ultrasonic lithotriptor is our choice for stone destruction, because it can evacuate stones simultaneously. A stone should be fragmented step by step from its periphery, taking care to avoid disintegrated stones escaping into the calices. If a stone is exceedingly hard, the use of a pneumatic lithotriptor (Lithocrast, EMS, Switzerland) may be recommended, although it is then a troublesome procedure to remove the stones. Currently, however, this seems to be the most powerful lithotriptor available.

The irrigation pressure should be adjusted to minimize absorption of the irrigating fluid while still suppressing venous bleeding, thus securing a clear visual field. The lowest pressure that preserves the visual field is usually the best. When an ultrasonic lithotriptor is used, higher pressure may be needed, and the intrapelvic pressure is then adjusted by changing the vacuum pressure appropriately.

Stones in the renal calices which are hard to reach with a rigid pyeloscope can be destroyed and extracted using a flexible fiber nephroscope and a laser or electrohydraulic lithotriptor (EHL). However, it should be noted that the movement of the fiberscope is often limited when it is mounted on a laser or EHL probe. At present, residual stones can be treated with ESWL, and therefore it is not necessary to use PNL for clearing all stones.

PNL in Difficult Conditions

Although, as described in the previous section, many of the difficult conditions that occur are the result of careless procedures, truly difficult cases are sometimes encountered, even by technically skilled operators. These truly difficult circumstances, as well as some secondarily induced conditions, are listed in Table 2.

TABLE 2. Difficult conditions for PNL

1. When the initial access to the collecting system fails

2. When the target calyx cannot be visualized clearly

3. When access to the calyx to be punctured is difficult
   (1) Presence of a simple cyst
   (2) High location of the kidney
   (3) Interposition of a visceral organ on the ideal tract
   (4) Bent tract

4. When the target calyx tends to escape from the puncture
   (1) Excessively mobile kidney
   (2) Presence of excess fat around the kidney
   (3) Thin and fibrotic renal cortex

5. When large stones fill the renal pelvis and calices, thus hindering the insertion of a guide wire or a dilator

When Initial Access to the Collecting System Fails

During the formation of a nephrostomy tract, a situation occasionally occurs when a single careless move results in serious complications. In our experience, the most frequent problem has been the advancement of the guide wire outside the urinary tract and, which makes matters worse, the tract dilation going ahead. As in cases where the punctured calyx is full of stones, the guide wire can easily go outside the calyx after it has reached the right place. Once this happens, repeating the procedure rarely results in a successful outcome. Precautions must always be taken to prevent such an event happening, or if it does, not to insert the guide wire too far in the wrong direction. First, in the initial puncture, the needle should enter the calyx along the medial surface of the stone. In this way, the guide wire will advance to the middle of the pelvis, and the chances of it going directly toward the wall of the pelvis are small. Second, the position of the guide wire should be carefully monitored. During the manipulation of the wire, there should be regular checks to confirm that it is located precisely within the urinary tract, as outlined by a retrograde contrast injection from an occlusion ureteral catheter. If the guide wire is accidentally inserted into the peripelvic space [5], i.e., just outside the serosa of the pelvic wall and inside the peripelvic adipose tissue, the renal pelvic wall will move with the movement of the guide wire. In this situation, it is easy to believe mistakenly that the guide wire is within the collecting system. Therefore, the location of the guide wire should be carefully checked using multidirectional images on fluoroscopy. If there is any doubt about the position of the guide wire, this should be checked before dilation of the tract takes place. In order to confirm that the guide wire is positioned correctly, the tract is dilated to 7 or 8F and a 5-F open-ended catheter is advanced over the wire. A small amount of contrast medium is then injected through the catheter. In cases where the catheter is not in the collecting system, the catheter is pulled back very slowly, and when its tip comes near the calyx, the catheter is suctioned to check for a possible backflow of urine. If urine backflow is observed, a contrast medium is injected to confirm that the catheter tip is within the collecting system. The guide wire is then inserted again, and routine procedures could be resumed to establish the tract. If this repeat procedure fails, a new puncture is recommended targeting a somewhat different portion of the same calyx. If a tract has already been dilated, the situation is more complicated. It must be realized that once a large perforation hole has been made, the reinserted guide wire would tend to go the wrong way. Therefore, it is prudent to limit the following procedures merely to placing the nephrostomy at this stage. After the formation of a false tract, echo-guided repuncture is extremely difficult, so it may be better to use a fluoroscopic image. Observation of the tract with a small caliber ureteroscope inserted along the guide wire is sometimes successful, and it is worth attempting to manipulate the guide wire under ureteroscopic visualization. These special cases in which a false tract develops are usually associated with a large stone, so fluoroscopic targeting of only the part of the stone corresponding to the calyx may be easier. Feeling a stone at the needle tip can be used as a sign of a successful puncture. Relying on that feeling, a guide wire should be negotiated along the stone on the opposite side to the false tract. The new tract should then be dilated to 14 or 16 F. The final procedure on that day should be to insert a single-J-indwelling catheter. There may be various other reasons for the failure of a puncture. It is important to find out the most likely reasons and to deal with those undesirable conditions. What must not be done is to make the situation worse. If contrast visualization is needed, as small an amount of the medium as possible should be injected. An external injection further blurs the targeting with both echo-guided and fluoroscopy-guided punctures. Figure 4 shows a case in which a false tract was created and an indwelling, single-J catheter was placed incorrectly. In this typical case, the guide wire entered the collecting system once, but then a further push against soft tissue resistance moved it outside. Pulling out the indwelling catheter relocated the catheter tip inside the collecting system.

When the Target Calyx Cannot Be Visualized Clearly

In general, fluoroscopy-guided puncture can be done more accurately than an echo-guided puncture because the process of stepwise advancement of the needle can be checked in real time. In this way, the direction and depth of the puncture are checked precisely. Moreover, the stone itself can be used as a target. Either the point on the stone or the point near the stone corresponding to the calyx can be targeted. In this case, a monitor should be placed so that the operator can coordinate the procedure according to the visual movements on the monitor. This use of an appropriately placed monitor is the same for laparoscopic handling.

As described above, the collecting system should be distended by an indwelling occlusion balloon in the ureter before the puncture. However, this preparation is

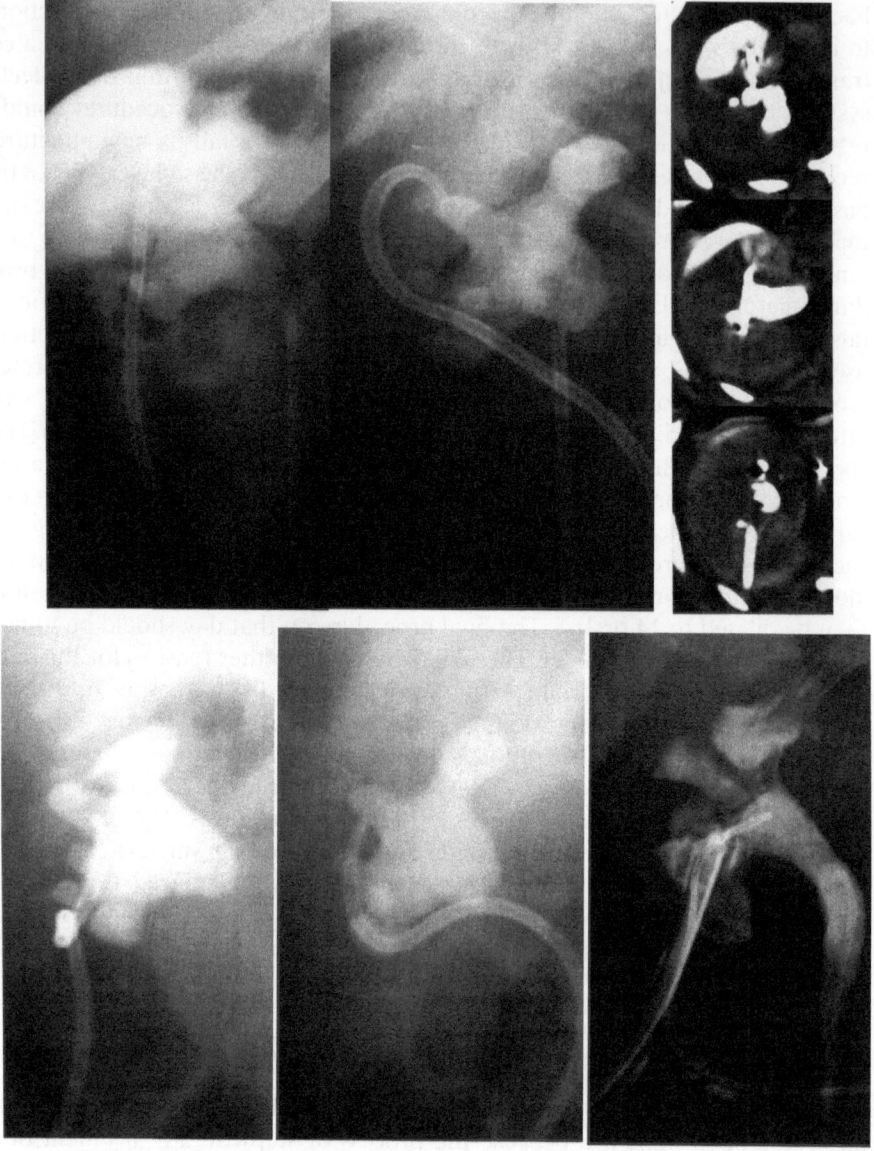

FIG. 4. A case with an incorrect location of the guide wire and catheter, followed by their relocation. The nephrostomy catheter was advanced outside the collecting system (*upper panel*). This was corrected by pulling the catheter back into the collecting system under fluoroscopic control (*lower panel*). It was confirmed that the tract was in the correct position by antegrade pyelography after PNL

sometimes precluded by factors such as prostatic hyperplasia, or a condition that has developed after uretrovesiconeostomy. Drip infusion pyelography with diuresis, or a pilot puncture of the most accessible calyx may be alternatives. If a small puncture needle is used and the tract is not dilated, the renal pelvis could be the target for a pilot puncture. When a pilot puncture of the calyx is successful, it is preferable to keep the tract and place an indwelling, small-size single-J catheter in it. A soft catheter will probably not disturbe the procedures needed to make an ideal tract. Visualization of the collecting system with a contrast injection through the pilot catheter may help in the creation of an ideal tract.

When a simple cyst located close to the target calyx blurs the echo-visualization of the calyx, it can be used as a landmark for the puncture, instead of considering it to be a disturbing factor. If the location of the target in relation to the cyst is understood in advance, the calyx could be punctured by piercing through the appropriate part of the cyst. If the needle tip only reaches the cyst, the fluid within the cyst can be suctioned out and the needle advanced 1 or 2 cm further. The rest of the procedure is the same as in conventional tract formation. Alternatively, the cyst can be treated in advance with an ethanol injection, and the treatment of the renal stone can wait until the cyst has healed.

When Access to the Ideal Calyx to be Punctured is Difficult

When the kidney is in a high position, a special procedure might be needed. An intercostal puncture should be avoided in patients with asthma or other pulmonary dysfunction. The position of the lower margin of the pleura should be confirmed by preoperative chest X-ray or CT in the prone position, especially during an inhalation phase. When the pleural margin is not particularly low, the intercostal space between the 11th and 12th ribs may be punctured without injuring the pleura as long as the puncture is done in the midinspiratory cycle or the exhalation phase, and is located at a considerably anterior site. A puncture during the deep inhalation phase should be avoided. With any intercostal puncture, however, possible injury to the pleura should always be considered. It is always recommended that a chest X-ray be taken following PNL. Even when nothing unusual has been noticed during the process of PNL, pneumothorax could become apparent at the time of withdrawal of the tract sheath. In such a case, the tract should be manually compressed and thoracic drainage should be carried out immediately. Although a two-tract approach has been reported [6], this method requires a special technique. At present, various supplementary instruments such as small-caliber fiberscopes, laser lithotriptors, and topical shockwave lithotriptors are available. If these newly developed instruments are used an easier and less invasive treatment can be chosen.

When the kidney position is high, a puncture of the middle calyx may be difficult to access even from the intercostal space. Thus, the lowermost calyx should be punctured in a deep inhalation phase, and the tract should also be dilated in the inhalation phase. Otherwise, the tract may be bent and elongated during the upward movement of the kidney. Since the line from the puncture site to the targeted lower calyx and that from the calyx to the renal pelvis are at an angle, a guide wire might not advance to the renal pelvis, and instead, coil itself in the calyx. In such a case, the use of a ureteroscope in the early stage of dilation may be recommended. After the tract has been dilated to 12 or 14 F, a ureteroscope is inserted over or beside the guide wire, and the latter is advanced toward the renal pelvis under direct vision. Dilation of the tract should be carried out up to, and not across, the calyx. Under these circumstances, a metal dilator is the best instrument for further dilation. It allows the tract to be dilated even when the target calyx is very small, and it also keeps the tract straight, minimizing the respiratory movement of the calyx.

When the ideal puncture is not possible because of an intervening visceral organ, the next ideal calyx has to be chosen for the puncture. The same technical procedures as those described above are needed for tract formation.

When the Puncture Target Tends to Escape from the Puncture Line

In very thin patients, an extremely mobile kidney often makes the puncture difficult. The needle tip should be advanced quickly before the target can move away. For dilation, it is essential to keep the guide wire straight while dilating the tract to 12 F. It may be useful to change the guide wire to a stiffer one during this procedure. Thereafter, the tract should be dilated with metal dilators while keeping the calyx anchored at its tip. Quick advancement of the dilator through the renal parenchyma may be necessary. The use of a flexible dilator may result in bending of the tract, as shown in Fig. 3.

When the renal parenchyma is extremely thin, the cortex moves away when the dilator comes into contact with the renal capsule. Therefore, the dilator will also need to be pushed quickly at the moment when it penetrates the cortex. During the dilation, the collecting system should always be visualized fluoroscopically.

When Large Stones Fill the Renal Collecting System and Hinder the Insertion of a Guide Wire and Dilators

When the renal pelvis is filled with staghorn calculi, the insertion of a guide wire in the pelvis as well as tract dilation become difficult. Although the space between the stone and the pelvic wall appears to be limited, it is usually distensible. Therefore, in many cases, a large-size dilator can be inserted without trouble. However, if the renal pelvic wall is fibrous and restricts these procedures, dilation of the tract up to the outer margin of the stone is recommended, and lithotripsy can be started from this point. Alternatively, the tract can be dilated to 17 F and the stone can be destroyed by a ureteroscopic instrument inserted through a small-size Amplatz sheath (Cook Urological, IN, USA).

Conclusion

Essentially, PNL is not difficult except when unusual anatomical hazards limit a percutaneous approach to the kidney. What makes PNL difficult is that neglect of the basic technical rules brings new complications. The essential thing for successful PNL is to understand the rationale of the basic technical principles and to follow them, and if unexpected problems occur, to try to minimize them before any serious harm is done.

References

1. Segura JW, Preminger GM, Assimos DG, Dretler SP, Kahn RI, Lingeman JE, Macaluso JN Jr, McCullough DL (1994) Nephrolithiasis clinical guidelines panel summary report on the management of staghorn calculi. J Urol 151:1648–1651
2. Wolf JS Jr, Clayman RV (1997) Percutaneous nephrolithotomy: what is its role in 1997. Urol Clin North Am 24:43–58
3. Sampio FJB (2000) Renal anatomy: endourologic consideration. Urol Clin North Am 27:585–607
4. Clayman RV, McDougall EM, Nakada SY (1998) Endourology of the upper urinary tract: percutaneous renal and ureteral procedures. In: Campbell's urology, 7th edn. Saunders, Philadelphia, pp 2789–2874
5. Gil-Vernet J (1965) New surgical concepts in removing renal calculi. Urol Int 20:255–288
6. Karlin GS, Smith AD (1989) Approaches to the superior calix: renal displacement technique and review of options. J Urol 142:774–777

Technology of Shockwave Lithotripsy

GEORGE K. CHOW[1] and STEVAN B. STREEM[2]

Summary. Shockwave lithotripsy was the result of a technical breakthrough by aerospace engineers at Dornier. Since then, the urologic treatment of stone disease has undergone a complete transformation from a field defined by open surgery to one defined by minimally invasive techniques.

There are many components that make up a lithotriptor, but the defining element is its energy source. We categorize these machines by the type of shockwave generator employed. Each type of generator has its own advantages and disadvantages. Unfortunately, no quantitative value of a shockwave generator can be correlated to its qualitative effect.

New technologies and ideas have transformed both the form and the function of lithotriptors, so that they bear little resemblance to the original HM-1 prototype. Ongoing research is attempting to improve extracorporeal shockwave lithotripsy (ESWL) in several different ways. Improvements in shockwave generation, shockwave measurement, and stone localization should result in increasingly efficient lithotripsy. The application of the time reversal process to lithotripsy will allow lithotriptors to track stones and electronically steer shock waves toward the target automatically. A reduction in cavitary fields may result in less pain.

Key Words. Endourology, Lithotripsy, Technology, Urolithiasis, Shock waves

Introduction

No single technology has changed the field of urology as much as shockwave lithotripsy (SWL). The first clinical application of SWL was reported by Chaussy et al. in 1980 [1]. During the next two decades, the urological management of

[1] Johns Hopkins Bayview Medical Center, 4940 Eastern Ave., Rm 344, Baltimore, MD 21224, USA
[2] Cleveland Clinic Foundation, 9500 Euclid Ave., A100, Cleveland, OH 44195, USA

nephrolithiasis has evolved from open surgery to noninvasive and minimally invasive techniques, and open stone surgery is rarely indicated today [2]. In this chapter, we discuss the basic technical components of SWL, compare the various lithotriptors, and explore the future of SWL in terms of recent developments.

Early detractors of SWL were concerned that the stone fragments created by lithotripsy would not be expelled by the body. However, Chaussy et al. [1] demonstrated in a canine model that effective fragment clearance was possible. Many clinicians were concerned about the potential for SWL-induced injury to the kidney and adjacent organs. Long-term studies have shown that it is both safe and efficacious [3–7].

Dornier, a German aerospace firm, discovered shockwave lithotripsy [8, 9]. Engineers at Dornier were studying the effects of shock waves generated by supersonic aircraft, and serendipitously observed the acoustic phenomenon that would lead to the first lithotriptor. In an effort to create reproducible and directed shock waves, an electrohydraulic or "spark gap" generator was developed. The HM-1 (human machine) was introduced on February 20, 1980 [1]. Within 4 years, the first available commercial lithotriptor, the HM-3, was on the market.

After the introduction of the HM-3, a second generation of lithotriptors was introduced during the mid-1980s. New energy sources such as the piezoelectric (1986) [10, 11] and electromagnetic (1987) [12] generators were introduced. Other innovations included the introduction of bath-less lithotriptors (1980), the use of ultrasound imaging (1985), and the replacement of general anesthesia with intravenous analgesia [9].

A "third" generation of lithotriptors has been developed to address the issue of cost [13]. With decreasing medical budgets, market pressure has induced the development of more compact and inexpensive machines.

Mechanics of Shockwave Lithotripsy

Lithotriptor operation can be divided into several key functional components.

1. Shockwave source.
2. Shockwave focusing.
3. Coupling.
4. Imaging.
5. Anesthesia.

Shockwave Source

Lithotriptors are usually categorized on the basis of their energy source. There are three forms of energy source in common use today. These include electrohydraulic, piezoelectric, and electromagnetic sources. Another experimental energy source is microexplosive, but there is no commercially available lithotriptor employing this type of generator.

Electrohydraulic lithotriptors were the first shockwave generators developed [1]. This energy source relies upon a spark-gap electrode to generate the shock waves. A high-voltage discharge from the electrode vaporizes water at the F_1 focal point. This gaseous expansion generates a shock wave that diverges from the point of origin until it hits an ellipsoid or parabolic reflector. The reflected waves are then redirected to a second focal point (F_2), where the stone is situated.

Further experimentation resulted in the discovery of the piezoelectric generator in 1986 [12]. With this type of generator, a hemispheric dish or receptacle is lined with piezoelectric crystals. When a high-voltage current is applied to the dish, the piezoelectric crystals expand simultaneously, generating a shock wave. The concave dish that houses the piezoelectric crystals is shaped in a way that permits the projection of the shock waves so that they converge at a focal point at which a calculus is targeted.

Use of a electromagnetic generator was first reported by Wilbert et al. in 1987 [11]. These lithotriptors employ a water-filled shock tube in which a metallic membrane is backed by a magnetic coil. When current is circulated in the coil, the resulting charge on the coil repels the oppositely charged metallic membrane. A shock wave is generated by this magnetic repulsion. An acoustic lens or parabolic reflector directs the shock wave to the targeted focal point.

Microexplosive generators have not met with commercial success. Kuwahara et al. [14] first described microexplosive generators in 1986. An explosion of tiny lead azide pellets generates shock waves. A parabolic reflector directs the shock wave to the F_2 focal point. Although effective, microexplosive generators have failed to come into widespread use owing to concerns about the storage and handling of the explosive lead azide pellets.

Shockwave Focusing

Shockwave focusing describes the mechanism used to direct and concentrate shockwave energy at the focal point. Each form of energy source has a unique mechanism of shockwave focusing. All of these methods rely on some form of lens or reflector to alter the direction of the shock waves. The critical attributes of a given focusing device are focal zone and aperture. The focal zone is the actual volume in which the shock waves are concentrated. The larger the focal zone, the higher the shockwave energy and peak pressure [5, 9]. Higher peak pressures result in more powerful stone fragmentation. Unfortunately, larger focal zones also result in more shockwave energy being delivered to surrounding body tissues, resulting in increased pain.

The shockwave aperture is the area of the acoustic lens, shock tube, or reflector, and roughly corresponds to the surface area of the skin penetrated by the shock waves. Piezoelectric lithotriptors, which have wide apertures, tend to have low energy density at the entry point of the shock waves through the skin. Lower cutaneous energy results in less pain for the patient [5, 10].

Coupling

Shockwave coupling refers to the medium transmitting the shock wave. Ideally, the medium should minimally dissipate the shockwave energy. A bath filled with gas-less water served as the coupling mechanism in the HM-3, the first commercial lithotriptor. Now, water cushions composed of material with appropriate acoustic properties are substituted for a water bath. Although "dry" lithotriptors appear to deliver less shockwave energy to the target, they are in widespread use owing to the ease of patient positioning, and the possibility of treating the patient in the prone position [9].

Imaging

The two imaging techniques used in SWL are fluoroscopy and ultrasonography. The first lithotripters relied on fluoroscopy to guide the shock wave. Although the dosage of radiation delivered during SWL is well within safe limits, ultrasonography has been an attractive alternative means of imaging [15]. As well as the obvious advantage of eliminating radiation exposure, the means to perform continuous real-time monitoring of treatment, and the possibility of treating radiolucent calculi are attractive features [9]. Unfortunately, ultrasonic image quality can suffer because of intervening bowel gas, and ureteral calculi are often invisible to ultrasound [9].

Anesthesia

Initially, SWL relied on a general or regional anesthetic. Subsequently, a number of techniques have been introduced to greatly simplify anesthesia. Intravenous sedation with sedative hypnotics such as midazolam, or short-acting narcotics such as fentanyl, have proved to be effective analgesic regimens for SWL [16]. Topical anesthetic agents such as EMLA cream have been shown to decrease the amount of intravenous agent required [9]. Topical vaseline has been shown to decrease the anesthetic requirement [17]. Vaseline's purported mechanism is that the viscosity of the vaseline prevents shockwave-induced cavitation at the skin level.

Whatever the method of anesthesia chosen, respiratory excursion can hinder effective shockwave delivery [18]. If increased shocks and more frequent patient repositioning are required, this can result in increased treatment time with resultant increases in radiation exposure [15, 19]. High-frequency jet ventilation was developed to minimize respiratory excursion during treatment [18, 19]. Although better fragmentation and shorter treatment times were obtained with this method, altering the rate or depth of ventilation to this degree compromised patient oxygenation. Owing to this untoward effect, this technique is no longer in use [20].

Comparison of Lithotriptors

The principal difference between the various models of lithotriptor available today is the form of energy source used. Electrohydraulic lithotriptors are advantageous owing to their larger focal points, flexible apertures, and moderately high peak pressures [7, 9, 21]. The disadvantages of an electrohydraulic energy source include a short functional life span and poorly reproducible shock waves. The lack of shockwave reproduciblity is derived from the alteration in the electrical current from positive to negative elements on the electrode, which occurs with increasing use [9, 22]. With electrode wear, the distance between the positive and negative tips can increase. The geometry of the ellipsoid reflector is such that a small alteration in this distance can result in dramatic changes in the width of the focal zone at F_2. Unfortunately, this phenomenon results in frequent electrode changes.

The advantages of a piezoelectric energy source are a long functional life span, superior patient comfort, and the ability to vary shockwave frequencies [7]. Piezoelectric lithotriptors have the widest apertures; this feature accounts for the decreased analgesia requirements [10]. Unfortunately, this characteristic also results in small focal zones. Although high-pressure pulses are sent to the focal zone, the actual energy density delivered is less owing to the small volume of the focal zone [9]. Because the focal zone is small, there is little margin of error when targeting a given calculus. Finally, piezoelectric generators suffer from the fact that they have a limited energy range.

Electromagnetic lithotriptors also have excellent functional longevity compared with electrohydraulic lithotriptors. They can deliver several hundred thousand shocks between services, thereby obviating the need continually to replace electrodes. Also, they have a wide and continuous gradation of energy settings. The disadvantages of these machines include the necessity to change the metallic membrane, albeit not very frequently [9].

Each energy source creates unique fragmentary patterns [23]. Electrohydraulic lithotriptors produce craters that are shallow and wide. Conversely, piezoelectric lithotriptors create narrow deep defects. Electromagnetic lithotriptors create craters shaped like a right-angled circular cone. With electrohydraulic and piezoelectric lithotriptors, maximal fragmentation is achieved by targeting the focal point on the anterior surface of the stone. Electromagnetic lithotriptors, on the other hand, work best with the focal point positioned on the posterior surface of the calculus. When the ability to target stones is more accurate, these properties can be applied clinically to improve stone fragmentation.

The differences between some common lithotriptors are summarized in Table 1.

TABLE 1. Comparison of some commonly used lithotriptors

Model	Manufacturer	Shockwave source	Focus	Coupling	Peak pressure (bars)	Stone localization	Max. focal zone W mm × L mm
HM-3	Dornier	Electrohydraulic	Ellipsoid	Water bath	1300	X-ray	15 × 90
MFL 5000	Dornier	Electrohydraulic	Ellipsoid	Water cushion	1000	X-ray/US	10 × 40
MPL 9000	Dornier	Electrohydraulic	Ellipsoid	Water cushion	1300	Coaxial X-ray/US	3 × 20
Nova	Direx	Electrohydraulic	Ellipsoid	Water cushion	N/A	X-ray	4 × 15
Econolith	Medispec	Electrohydraulic	Ellipsoid	Water cushion	725	X-ray	13 × 53
Sonolith 3000	Technomed	Electrohydraulic	Ellipsoid	Minibath	1000	US	15 × 55
STS	Medstone	Electrohydraulic	Ellipsoid	Water cushion	350	X-ray/US	13 × 50
Compact	Dornier	Electromagnetic	Acoustic lens	Water cushion	460	Lateral US/X-ray	6.4 × 70
Do Li S	Dornier	Electromagnetic	Acoustic lens	Water cushion	715	X-ray	3.8 × 49.2
Lithostar Plus	Siemens	Electromagnetic	Acoustic lens	Water cushion	650	X-ray/coaxial US	4 × 40
Modulith	Storz	Electromagnetic	Parabolic	Water cushion	1000	X-ray/coaxial US	6 × 30
LT01	Edap	Piezoelectric	Spherical dish	Water cushion	1144	Coaxial US	5 × 23
LT02	Edap	Piezoelectric	Spherical dish	Water cushion	1400	X-ray/coaxial US	1.8 × 29
Piezolith 2300	Wolf	Piezoelectric	Concave dish	Minibath	1200	Coaxial US	2.5 × 30
Piezolith 2500	Wolf	Piezoelectric	Concave dish	Water cushion	1200	X-ray/coaxial US	1.5 × 11

N/A, not applicable; US, ultrasound.

Future Developments

Shockwave Energy

Methods are being developed to augment shockwave energy. Broyer et al. [22] describe the use of a "coaxial discharge line" to improve the electroacoustic efficiency of the electrohydraulic lithotriptor. Increasing the electroacoustic efficiency will mean that the same fragmentation efficiency can be achieved with a lower treatment voltage. This should decrease patient discomfort and extend the life of the electrodes. Interestingly, increasing the focal energy density does not always result in improved fragmentation. Vandeursen et al. [24] compared high- and low-pressure electromagnetic lithotriptors and failed to notice any improvement in fragmentation with increased pressure.

Reduction of Cavitary Fields

As has been explained previously, electrohydraulic lithotriptors rely on a reflector to focus shock waves toward the F_2 focal point. Bailey et al. [25] have discovered that replacing rigid reflectors with pressure-release reflectors can stifle bubble growth, and thereby reduce cavitation intensity. Since pain from treatment is felt to derive from cavitation at the skin level, perhaps cavitation reduction will lead to more patient comfort. However, at this stage, this technical innovation is reserved for experimental observations of the role of cavitation in lithotripsy.

Clinical Shockwave Measurement

Acoustic hydrophones have been employed to analyze shock waves in the laboratory setting. The miniaturization of this technology has permitted the creation of retrograde ureteral probes for the continuous measurement of shock waves during treatment [26]. Currently, there is no clinical application for such technology, since pressure measurements do not always correlate with treatment efficacy. Buizza et al. [5] have examined the pulse pressures generated by a number of different lithotriptors, and concluded that "it is difficult or even impossible to relate the ESWL pressure field parameters with treatment effectiveness." Nevertheless, Coleman et al. [26] believe that in situ acoustic measurements will have a clinical impact. It is postulated that this technology will allow urologists to maximize treatment energy within defined acoustic safety parameters.

Radiographic Improvement

SWL efficacy is highly dependent on accurate imaging. Swanson [27] has described the technique of intraoperative excretory urography to facilitate stone targeting, especially for radiolucent calculi. Pearle et al. [28] compared bolus injection and drip infusion of contrast during SWL. A statistically significant reduction in imaging time and contrast volume employed was noted when bolus injection was employed instead of drip infusion.

Real-Time Calculus Targeting

As mentioned previously, renal movement during respiratory excursion is a significant impediment to accurate stone targeting. Synchronization of shock waves to the respiratory cycle has been explored [29]. Another strategy relies on a second piezoelectric array as a low-amplitude transmitter. Pulse echo signals that return from the stone would show a high amplitude if that stone was located at the focus. This high-amplitude signal would in turn trigger a shock wave [30]. Another intriguing technique relies on storage of the ultrasound image of the calculus on computer [31]. Shock waves are only triggered when the same ultrasound image is seen in the focal zone. However, even though these techniques do decrease the number of shocks needed to disintegrate a stone, they also take up considerably more time [32]. A more promising technology is time-reversal focusing or electronic beam steering [32, 33]. This technique utilizes the "time reversal" phenomenon to allow for continuous tracking of a target calculus. Thomas et al. [33] describe the time reversal process as "[detecting] the ultrasonic pressure field generated by an active acoustic source (i.e., calculus) embedded in a heterogeneous medium with a set of transducer elements. The signal received by each element is digitized and recorded during a time interval T. These sampled signals are then read in a reversed temporal chronology and retransmitted by the same transducers. It has been shown that this time reversal process enables the transducer array to focus on the source location." Cathignol et al. [32] demonstrated that electronic focusing permits calculus tracking over an ellipsoid region of $4\,cm \times 6\,cm$.

Conclusions

The serendipitous discovery of shockwave lithotripsy has dramatically affected the field of urology. It has heralded an era of minimally invasive urology. Open stone surgery, once so common, is now a rarity. This trend away from open surgery has benefited patients by less postoperative pain, shorter hospital stays, and more rapid convalescence.

As we have seen, the lithotriptor is often defined by the source of shockwave energy employed. Each form of shockwave generation has its inherent advantages and disadvantages. Interestingly, they each have a unique fragmentation "fingerprint." In today's healthcare environment, the focus of lithotriptor development has shifted toward economy; smaller and less expensive third-generation lithotriptors are coming onto market.

Several new technologies are being developed to enhance shockwave lithotripsy. Improvements in shockwave generation and focusing may result in more effective and less painful lithotripsy. The efficacy of lithotripsy may be enhanced by the development of acoustic probes that can direct the application of shock waves. Furthermore, calculus targeting technology could be enhanced and automated to such an extent that the urologist may not even need to be present.

Shockwave lithotripsy is a revolutionary technology that has transformed the specialty of urology. As with many discoveries, serendipity played an important role. We are fortunate that the engineers at Dornier were perceptive enough to recognize the significance of their discovery.

References

1. Chaussy C, Brendel W, Schmiedt E (1980) Extracorporeally induced destruction of kidney stones by shock waves. Lancet 2:1265–1268
2. Paik ML, Wainstein MA, Spirnak JP, et al. (1998) Current indications for open stone surgery in the treatment of renal and ureteral calculi. J Urol 159:374–379
3. Begun FP, Lawson RK, Kearns CM, Tieu TM (1989) Electrohydraulic shock wave induced renal injury. J Urol 142:155–159
4. Bierkens AF, Hendrikx VJW, DeKort T, et al. (1992) Efficacy of second generation lithotripters: a multicenter comparative study of 2206 ESWL treatments with the Siemens lithostar, Dornier HM-4, Wolf piezolith 2300, Direx tripter X-1 and Breakstone lithotripters. J Urol 148:1052–1057
5. Biuzza A, Dell'Aquilla T, Giribona P (1995) The performance of different pulse pressure generators for extracorporeal lithotripsy: a comparison based on commercial lithotripters for kidney stones. Ultrasound Med Biol 21:259–272
6. Ehreth JT, Drach GW, Arnett ML, et al. (1994) Extracorporeal shock wave lithotripsy: multicenter study of kidney and upper ureter versus middle and lower ureter treatments. J Urol 152:1379–1385
7. Thomas VM, Sosa RE (1998) Shock wave lithotripsy. In: Walsh PC, Retik AB, Vaughn ED, Wein AJ (eds) Campbell's urology. 7th edn. Saunders, Philadelphia
8. Jocham D (1987) Historical development of ESWL. In: Riehle RA (ed) Principles of extracorporeal shock wave lithotripsy. Churchill Livingstone, New York, pp 1–11
9. Lingeman JE (1997) ESWL: development, instrumentation and current status. Urol Clin N Am 24:185–211
10. Marberger M, Turk C, Steinkogler I (1988) Painless piezoelectric extracorporeal lithotripsy. J Urol 139:695–699
11. Wilbert DM, Richenberger H, Noske E, et al. (1987) New generation shock wave lithotripsy. J Urol 138:563–565
12. Thibault PH, Dory J, Cotard JP, et al. (1988) Lithotripsie a impulsions ultra-courtes: etude experimentale sur une lithiase renale du chien. Ann Urol 20:20–25
13. Lingeman JE (1995) Update on ESWL. AUA Update 14(28):226–231
14. Kuwahara M, Kambe K, Kurosu S, et al. (1997) Clinical application of ESWL using microexplosions. J Urol 137:837–840
15. VanSwearingen FL, McCullough DL, Dyer R, Appel B (1987) Radiation exposure to patients during ESWL. J Urol 138:18–20
16. Zonnick J, Leveillee R, Zabbo A, et al. (1996) Comparison of general anesthesia and intravenous sedation-analgesia for shock wave lithotripsy. J Endourol 10:489–491
17. Heidenreich A, jBonfig R, Wilbert DM, Engelmann UH (1995) Painless ESWL by cutaneous application of vaseline. Scand J Urol Nephrol 29:155–160

18. Whelan JP, Gravensten N, Welch I, et al. (1988) Simulation of ventilator induced stone movement and its effects on stone fracture during extracorporeal shock wave lithotripsy. J Urol 140:405–407

19. Warner MA, Warner ME, Buck CF, Segura JW (1988) Clinical efficiency of high frequency jet ventilation during ESWL of renal and ureteral calculi: a comparison with conventional mechanical ventilation. J Urol 139:486–487

20. Berger JJ, Boysen PG, Gravensten JS, et al. (1987) Failure of high frequency jet ventilation to ventilate patients adequately during ESWL. Anesth Analg 66:262–263

21. Hunter PT, Finlayson B, Hirko RJ, et al. (1986) Measurement of shock wave pressures used for lithotripsy. J Urol 136:733–738

22. Broyer P, Cathignol D, Theillere Y, et al. (1996) High efficiency shock wave generation for extracorporeal lithotripsy. Med Biol Eng Comput 34:321–328

23. Chuong CJ, Zhong P, Preminger GM (1992) A comparison of stone damage caused by different modes of shock wave generation. J Urol 148:200–205

24. Vandeursen H, DeRidder D, Pittomvils G, et al. (1993) High pressure vs. low pressure electromagnetic extracorporeal lithotripsy. J Urol 149:988–991

25. Bailey MR, Blackstock DT, Cleveland RO, et al. (1999) Comparison of electrohydraulic lithotripters with rigid and pressure-release ellipsoidal reflectors. II. Cavitary fields. J Acoust Soc Am 106(2):1149–1159

26. Coleman AJ, Draquioti E, Tiptaf R, et al. (1998) Acoustic performance and clinical use of a fiberoptic hydrophone. Ultrasound Med Biol 24:143–151

27. Swanson SK (1992) Excretory urography during ESWL: a localization alternative. Urology 39:185–186

28. Pearle MS, McClennen BL, Roehrbon CG, Clayman RV (1997) Bolus injection vs. drip contrast administration for ureteral stone targeting during shock wave lithotripsy. J Endourol 11:163–166

29. Ishida A (1989) Apparatus for destroying calculuses. Patent No. 0336620A2

30. Ishida A (1991) Lithotripsy apparatus having a missed-shot prevention function. Patent No. 0461479A1

31. Dawson C, Corry DA, Bowsher WG, et al. (1996) Use of image enhancement during lithotripsy. J Endourol 10:335–339

32. Cathignol D, Birer A, Nachef S, et al. (1995) Electronic beam steering of shock waves. Ultrasound Med Biol 21:365–377

33. Thomas JL, Wu F, Fink M (1996) Time reversal focusing applied to lithotripsy. Ultrasonic Imaging 18:106–121

Ureteroscopic Lithotripsy

MICHAEL GRASSO III

Summary. Endoscopic lithotripsy is based on direct visualization and fragmentation of a calculus within the urinary tract. The development of small-diameter fiberoptic endoscopes and various energy forms employed for fragmentation has facilitated retrograde, ureteroscopic treatment of many upper urinary tract calculi. Stones within the ureter and intrarenal calculi can be accessed and fragmented with this instrumentation. Specifically, 2.5-mm semirigid endoscopes are used in the most distal ureter, while flexible, actively deflectable ureteroscopes are employed in the proximal collecting system. Endoscopic lithotrites have progressed from ultrasound and electrohydraulic shockwave generators to laser lithotriptors. The holmium laser represents the most recent addition. This device actually converts stones to fine dust and small fragments, which frequently pass spontaneously from the collecting system after therapy. In general, the combination of contemporary endoscopes and the holmium laser lithotriptor can facilitate successful treatment of the majority of urinary calculi irrespective of size, location, and composition.

Key Words. Ureteroscopy, Calculi, Lithotripsy, Holmium laser

Smaller Diameter, Refined Ureteroscopes and Progressive Endoscopic Lithotriptors

In 1983, a group at the University of Chicago described the complementary use of rigid and the actively deflectable, flexible ureteroscopes [1]. The rigid endoscopes were employed in the distal half of the ureter, while the flexible endoscopes addressed more proximal ureteral and even intrarenal lesions. The flexible ureteroscopes were steerable, and in addition had a working channel that allowed deflectable lithotripsy probes (e.g., electrohydraulic) to be placed onto calculi for

NYU Medical Center, Department of Urology, New York University School of Medicine, 540 First Avenue, Suite 10U, New York, NY 10016, USA fragmentation. It was this complementary use of endoscopes that allowed the efficient treatment of many upper urinary tract stone burdens, often irrespective of size and location.

Endoscope miniaturization began initially with rigid ureteroscopes. The first endoscopes in this class were based on rod lens imaging, and ranged from 10 to 12 F in diameter. The application of fiberoptics in a stainless steel cylinder produced a semirigid endoscope which was miniaturized to 7 F, had standard working channel(s), and could be passively deflected in the ureter while maintaining a clear optical image. These endoscopes replaced the larger rigid ureteroscopes, and occasionally required intramural ureteral dilation for access [2, 3].

Actively deflectable, flexible ureteroscope miniaturization was the product of smaller fiberoptic bundles and modifications of internal design which led to a standard 7.5 F tip with a 3.6 F working channel [4]. Current flexible endoscope specifications by manufacturers are given in Table 1. With outer miniaturization, the diameter of the single working channel has been maintained. Two-way active tip deflection and secondary deflection, which is a weakness in a specific area on the proximal end of the endoscope, allow the dependant lower pole calyx to be inspected and lesions within it treated.

The smaller ureteroscopes are currently employed not only for endoscopic lithotripsy, but also for treating urothelial lesions, including upper urinary tract papillary tumors, ureteral and intrarenal strictures, and UPJ stenosis [5]. With this expansion in applications, the major complication rate when employing these

TABLE 1. Small diameter actively deflectable, flexible ureteroscopes: specifications [5]

	Manufacturer				
	Storz	Acmi	Wolf	Mitsubishi	Olympus
Model	11274AA	AUR 7	7325.171	971101	URF-P2Y
Diameter (F)					
Distal end	7.5	7.4	7.5	7.9	6.9/8.4
Body	8.2	7.5	7.5	7.9	8.4
Optics					
Field of view (°)	70	80	60	70	90
Angle of view (°)	0	12	0	0	0
Depth of focus (mm)	2–50	2–50	3–30	3.5	1.7–50
Optical bundle	Standard	Standard	Fused quartz	Fused quartz	Standard
Pixels per bundle	3000	3400	5000	6000	5500
Working channel diameter (F)	3.6	3.6	3.6	3.6	3.6
Deflection					
Active deflection (down/up in degrees)	170/120	160/120	160/130	134/170	100/180
Logical deflection (thumb lever down = tip down)	+	+	+	+	–
Secondary deflection	+	+	+	+	+

TABLE 2. Comparison of complication rates associated with ureteroscopy. There is a noticeable decrease in the major complication rates with greater experience and endoscope miniaturization

Author	Blute et al. [8]	Abdel-Razzak and Bagley [7]	Harmon et al. [6]	Grasso and Bagley [5]
Year published	1988	1992	1997	1998
Procedures	346	290	209	584
Minor complication				
Colic/pain (%)	–	9.0	3.5	5.5
Fever (%)	6.2	6.9	2.0	1.4
False passage (%)	0.9	–	–	0.4
Hematuria				
Minor (%)	0.5	2.1	0	0.7
Prolonged (%)	0.3	1.0	0	0.2
Extravasation (%)	0.6	1.0	–	–
UTI (%)	–	1.0	–	1.6
Pyelonephritis (%)	–	–	–	0.5
Major complications				
Perforation (%)	4.6	1.7	1.0	0
Stricture (%)	1.4	0.7	0.5	0.5
Avulsion (%)	0.6	0	0	0
Urinoma (%)	0.6	–	0	0
Urosepsis (%)	0.3	0	0	0
CVA (%)	–	–	0.5	0.2
DVT (%)	–	–	–	0.2

UTI, urinary tract infection; CVA, cerebrovascular accident; DVT, deep venous thrombasis.

instruments has actually decreased (Table 2) [5–8]. This is felt to be a product of the less traumatic insertion of the smaller-diameter endoscopes and improved surgical techniques.

Endoscopic lithotrites are instruments employed through the ureteroscope's working channel which fragment stone, often into extractable pieces. Baskets and endoscopic graspers are employed either to extract small calculi, or in a complementary role to decrease stone mobility during lithotripsy and remove fragments and debris created by this process. Ultrasonic lithotripsy was employed with the earliest rigid ureteroscopes. These probes loose power with either active or passive deflection, and as such are not complementary with contemporary endoscopes. Electrohydraulic probes were the first flexible endoscopic lithotriptors. These devices deliver energy circumferentially, which may damage adjacent tissue. In addition, EHL frequently fails to fragment the hardest calculi, including calcium oxalate monohydrate [9]. Pneumatic mechanical devices (i.e., lithoclasts) are small endoscopic jackhammers that work best when passed through a straight working channel. Employing reusable stainless steel probes through a semirigid ureteroscope, the lithoclast can efficiently and economically fragment calculi in the distal half of the ureter [10]. The application of a similar pneumatic stone jackhammer employed through a flexible ureteroscope has been reported

[11], and is based on the application of flexible nickel titanium probes. The mechanical pneumatic devices produce relatively large stone fragments that require extraction, and with particularly hard calculi, preventing stone migration during treatment can be challenging.

Laser lithotripsy began clinically in the 1980s with the coumarin-based pulsed-dye laser, which employs 504 nm of light delivered through optical quartz fibers [12]. This is a nonthermal laser which produces a plasma between the fiber's tip and the calculus, and fragments stone with a photoacoustic effect. The small flexible quartz probes were complementary to both the semirigid and the flexible ureteroscopes and could fragment most urinary calculi, excluding cystine. This was not, however, a solid-state laser, and required frequent maintenance. In addition, this wavelength fragmented the hardest stones into irregular shapes that often required endoscopic extraction. Finally, the energy available at the fiber's tip was limited by the fiber diameter [13]. The 200 micron fiber which restricted endoscopic deflection the least could only deliver 80 MJ energy. This was often insufficient to fragment calcium oxalate monohydrate calculi. For these reasons, the pulsed-dye laser has been replaced by more powerful, solid-state devices.

The holmium: yttrium–aluminum–garnet (YAG) laser is a thermal laser employing 2150 nm wavelength of light delivered in a pulsatile fashion through low water density quartz fibers. This device represents the most powerful of the endoscopic lithotrites employed to date. Johnson et al. [14] studied the soft tissue effects of this laser and found that within water, the thermal effect was confined owing to a vaporization bubble which formed at fiber's tip. In 1995, Matsuoka et al. [15] presented the first clinical series of endoscopic lithotripsy with this wavelength, and reported it to be safe and efficient in treating ureteral stones. As opposed to the pulsed-dye instruments, holmium laser lithotripsy produces fine dust and small fragments that can be at least partially irrigated from the collecting system during treatment [16]. When using the holmium laser, the energy available at the tip is not limited by the fiber's diameter, particularly when clinically useful energies are employed. Techniques have been developed to increase treatment efficiency by varying the laser fiber diameter with the endoscopes employed [17].

Pei Zhong et al. [18], at Duke University, carefully studied the effect of holmium laser energy on phantom stones and found that this specific wavelength fragments stones to fine dust and small particulate debris better than the other more standard lithotrites that were employed previously. This work also confirmed the clinical finding that by varying the energy delivered and the frequency of pulsation, stone mobility can be minimized while increasing the overall efficiency of treatment [19]. Defined clinically, the most efficient technique with this laser energy is to fragment stones down to fine dust and small debris rather than creating large pieces of stone that require actual endoscopic extraction to complete the treatment. One area of concern raised by Teichman et al. [20], from San Antonio, Texas, was the fact that holmium laser treatment of uric acid calculi can produce small amounts of cyanide. Initial laboratory studies were then expanded with a multicenter clinical trial where this was found to be of minimal clinical significance [21]. In general, long-term complications from holmium laser lithotripsy, and specifically the subsequent ureteral stricture rate, have been particularly low with contemporary techniques [22].

Progression of Ureteroscopic Lithotripsy from Ureteral to Intrarenal Calculi

Ureteroscopic lithotripsy, once felt to be indicated only for distal ureteral calculi, has been successfully employed in the more proximal upper urinary tract. The report by Erhard et al. [23] of a large series of proximal ureteral stones that were treated in a retrograde endoscopic fashion defined a success rate with contemporary techniques that approached 100%. Recent series also addressed the use of the actively deflectable, flexible ureteroscope and holmium lasers to treat intrarenal calculi. Fabrizio et al. [24] was able to completely fragment intrarenal calculi in 89% of 100 patients studied. The majority of these patients had failed prior shockwave lithotripsy, and for various reasons were either not candidates for or refused standard percutaneous nephrostolithotomy. Grasso and Chalik [25] presented success rates for ureteropyeloscopic lithotripsy stratified to specific ureteral and intrarenal locations. In this series, the largest calculi often required staged therapy, with the lower pole location having the lowest success (Table 3).

Flexible ureteroscopic access to the lower pole calyx is one of the most difficult manuevers when performing upper urinary tract endoscopy. In two-thirds of kidneys studied in one series, secondary endoscope deflection was required to place the flexible endoscope's tip into the lower pole [5]. The success rates for endoscopic lithotripsy when treating lower pole calculi stratified to intrarenal

TABLE 3. Retrograde ureteropyeloscopic treatment of ureteral and intrarenal calculi with the holmium:YAG laser [25]

Site	No. of stones	Mean diameter (mm) and range	Success rates (%)	
			Single session	Staged treatment
Ureter				
Proximal third	33	9.5 (23–25)	100	–
Middle third	29	12.7 (60–65)	97	100
Distal third	44	10.2 (50–55)	96	100
Totals	106		97	100
Intrarenal				
Upper pole	25	10.8 (35–34)	92	100
Middle pole	14	11.2 (23–24)	86	93
Lower pole	45	13.5 (40–43)	73	84
Renal pelvic	15	21.4 (60–66)	73	87
Totals	99		80	90

anatomical variants were studied by Elbahnasy et al. [26]. It was their conclusion that an acute infundibulopelvic angle and a long lower pole infundibulum affected the outcome of extracorporeal shockwave lithotripsy (ESWL) more than ureteroscopic lithotripsy in this setting. Grasso and Ficazzola [27] also reviewed their experience with endoscopic lithotripsy of lower pole intrarenal calculi. In their series they described techniques where endoscopic tools (i.e., graspers, etc.) were employed to move lower pole stones to more cephalad intrarenal locations where they could be treated more efficiently with a laser lithotriptor. The only two statistically significant variables of intrarenal anatomy which impacted negatively on treatment in this series were a lower pole infundibular length which exceeded 3 cm, or the presence of infundibular stenosis.

The treatment of large intrarenal stone burdens has traditionally been performed with percutaneous endoscopic techniques. Stones in excess of 2 cm, and in additon noninfectious staghorn calculi, treated with progressive ureteroscopic techniques have recently been reported [28]. In a multicenter trial, many patients who suffered from comorbid medical conditions, including bleeding diathesis, and who were not ideal candidates for traditional percutaneous nephrostolithotomy underwent ureteroscopic treatment. All calculi were in excess of 2 cm, with the maximum being a cystine stone burden 6 cm in longest diameter. Staged endoscopic therapy was required to treat the largest calculi because the fine dust and debris created by the holmium laser eventually obscured the optical field during treatment. The largest stone burdens ($\geqslant 3$ cm) frequently required a second-stage endoscopy to complete the treatment. Many of the procedures were performed under regional anesthetic and operative time approached 3 h for the most complex presentation. Operative success, defined as pulverizing the entire stone burden to fine dust and $\leqslant$ 2-mm fragments, was noted in the majority of patients studied. Follow-up imaging defined clearance of the fine dust and debris produced by holmium:YAG laser lithotripsy in 63% of patients, while small residual fragments were noted in 22%. Subsequent new stone growth was noted in only 15% of patients, and these had either uncorrectable metabolic disorders or intrarenal urinary stasis. There were no long-term complications at the three study sites, and specifically, postoperative ureteral strictures were not defined on follow-up imaging.

What is the Correct Treatment for Upper Urinary Tract Calculi: Ureteroscopic Versus Extracorporeal Shockwave Lithotripsy?

Both endoscopic and extracorporeal shockwave lithotripsy of upper urinary tract calculi became treatment options in the early 1980s. Ureteroscopy began with rigid endoscopes treating only distal ureteral stones [29]. ESWL was initially introduced as a treatment for uncomplicated, moderately sized renal calculi [30].

The indications for both treatments broadened over the next 15 years with improved instrumentation and imaging. The indications for ureteroscopic lithotripsy progressed up the ureter and then into the kidney with the application of the actively deflectable, flexible ureteroscope. Extracorporeal shockwave lithotriptors also evolved to second- and third-generation devices which had improved imaging, allowing for the treatment of ureteral stones, and less anesthetic requirements based on new generators with smaller focal zones [31]. These extracorporeal lithotriptors allowed easier localization, particularly of ureteral stones, and therefore there was great enthusiasm for treating all calculi throughout the entire upper urinary tract with this modality. However, the newest shockwave lithotriptors did not obtain the success rates of the first-generation Dornier HM3, which was in part secondary to broader treatment indications and the application of lower-power generators [32].

A polarization of thought supporting shockwave lithotripsy monotherapy (i.e., without ureteral stenting) for all stones throughout the upper urinary tract began in the early 1990s. A series of ESWL failures [33] were then followed by guidelines for treating upper urinary tract calculi. The first guidelines panel [34] dealt with the treatment of large renal stones (in excess of 2.5 cm). Percutaneous nephrostolithotomy was defined as a superior treatment in this setting, and shockwave lithotripsy monotherapy was contraindicated in most cases of large intrarenal calculi. The second guidelines panel addressed the treatment of ureteral calculi [35], and stratified stones based on size, location, and other concurrent findings, including ureteral obstruction. Ureteral calculi that were less than 5 mm in longest diameter, and not associated with high-grade upper urinary tract obstruction, will usually be passed without surgical intervention, and patients should be followed clinically unless prolonged, complete upper urinary tract obstruction or associated infection is defined. Larger ureteral calculi and those associated with significant obstruction can be treated either with ESWL or ureteroscopic lithotripsy. Both modalities were felt to be safe and effective. Shockwave lithotripsy based on the newest extracorporeal lithotriptors, is obviously less invasive than ureteroscopy, but may also be less efficacious than definitive endoscopic lithotripsy where fragment clearance may not be prompt or can be associated with secondary obstruction [40].

Conclusion

Treatment of upper urinary tract calculi is evolving based on improvements in ureteroscopic equipment and techniques, as well as the addition of second- and third-generation extracorporeal shockwave lithotriptors. Uncomplicated, moderately sized renal calculi continue to respond well to ESWL monotherapy. When broad indications for treatment are employed, however, the success rate reported with newer generation shockwave lithotriptors is lower. Ureteroscopic lithotripsy is obviously the next therapy for the majority of ESWL failures. In addition, with a success rate that approaches 100% in the ureter, ureteroscopy should be considered a first-line therapy in this setting. This is particularly true if a clinical presentation is complicated by large stone size, complete ureteral obstruction, etc. Finally, the beauty of ESWL is that it requires minimal anesthetic and is virtually noninvasive. If a ureteral catheter or retrograde stone manipulation is required under a regional or general anesthetic to enhance ESWL, ureteropyeloscopic lithotripsy, with its definitive nature and exceptionally high success rate, should be considered.

References

1. Bagley DH, Huffman JL, Lyon ES (1983) Combined rigid and flexible ureteropyeloscopy. J Urol 130:243–244
2. Stoller ML, Wolf JS Jr, Hofmann RS, Marc B (1992) Ureteroscopy without routine balloon dilation: an outcome assessment. J Urol 147:1238–1242
3. Abdel-Razzak O, Bagley DH (1993) The 6.9 F semi-rigid ureteroscope in clinical use. Urology 41:45–48
4. Grasso M, Bagley D (1994) A 7.5/8.2 F actively deflectable, flexible ureteroscope: a new device for both diagnostic and therapeutic upper urinary tract endoscopy. Urology 43:435–441
5. Grasso M, Bagley D (1998) Small diameter, actively deflectable, flexible ureteropyeloscopy. J Urol 160:1648–1654
6. Harmon WJ, Serson PD, Blute ML, et al. (1997) Ureteroscopy: current practice and long-term complications. J Urol 157:28–32
7. Abdel-Razzak OM, Bagley DH (1992) Clinical experience with flexible ureteropyeloscopy. J Urol 148:1788–1792
8. Blute ML, Segura JW, Patterson DE (1988) Uretroscopy. J Urol 139:510–512
9. Teichman JMH, Rao RD, Rogenes VJ, Harris JM (1997) Ureteroscopic management of ureteral calculi: electrohydraulic versus holmium:YAG lithotripsy. J Urol 158:1357–1364
10. Denstedt JD, Eberwein PM, Singh RR (1992) The Swiss lithoclast: a new device for intracorporeal lithotripsy. J Urol 148:1088–1090
11. Tawfiek ER, Grasso M, Bagley DH (1997) The initial use of the Browne pneumatic impactor. J Endourol 11:121–124
12. Dretler SP, Watson G, Parrish JA, Murray S (1987) Pulsed dye laser fragmentation of ureteral calculi: initial clinical experience. J Urol 137:386–389
13. Grasso M, Shalaby M, el Akkad M, Bagley D (1991) Techniques in endoscopic lithotripsy using the pulsed dye laser. Urology 37:138–144
14. Johnson DF, Cromeens DM, Price RE (1992) Use of the holmium:YAG laser in urology. Lasers Surg Med 12:353–363
15. Matsuoka K, Iida S, Nakanami M, et al. (1996) Holmium:yttrium–aluminium–garnet laser for endoscopic lithotripsy. Urology 45:947–952
16. Teichman JMH, Vassar GJ, Bishoff JT, Bellman GC (1998) Holmium:YAG lithotripsy yields smaller fragments than lithoclast, pulsed dye laser, or electrohydraulic lithotripsy. J Urol 159:17–23
17. Grasso M (1996) Experience with the holmium laser as an endoscopic lithotrite. Urology 48:199–206
18. Zhong P, Tong HL, Cocks FH, et al. (1998) Transient cavitation and acoustic emission produced by different laser lithotripters. J Endourol 12:371–378

19. Kuo RL, Aslan P, Zhong P, Preminger GM (1998) Impact of holmium laser settings and fiber diameter on stone fragmentation and endoscope deflection. J Endourol 12:523–527
20. Teichman JMH, Vassar GJ, Glickman RD, et al. (1998) Holmium:YAG lithotripsy: photothermal mechanism converts uric acid calculi to cyanide. J Urol 160:320–324
21. Teichman JMH, Champion PC, Wollin TA, Denstedt JD (1998) Holmium:YAG lithotripsy of uric acid calculi. J Urol 160:2130–2132
22. Beaghler M, Poon M, Ruckle H, et al. (1998) Complications employing the holmium:YAG laser. J Endourol 12:533–535
23. Erhard M, Salwen J, Bagley DH (1996) Ureteroscopic removal of mid- and proximal ureteral calculi. J Urol 155:38–42
24. Fabrizio MD, Behari A, Bagley DH (1998) Ureteroscopic management of intrarenal calculi. J Urol 159:1139–1143
25. Grasso M, Chalik Y (1998) Principles and applications of laser lithotripsy: experience with the holmium laser lithotrite. J Clin Laser Med Surg 16:3–7
26. Elbahnasy AM, Shalhav AL, Hoenig DM, et al. (1998) Lower caliceal stone clearance after shock wave lithotripsy or ureteroscopy: the impact of lower pole radiographic anatomy. J Urol 159:676–682
27. Grasso M, Ficazzola M (1999) Retrograde ureteropyeloscopic treatment of lower pole calyceal calculi. J Urol 162:1904–1908
28. Grasso M, Conlin M, Bagley D (1998) Retrograde ureteropyeloscopic treatment of 2 cm or greater upper urinary tract and minor staghorn calculi. J Urol 160:346–351
29. Chaussy C, Fuchs G, Kahr R, et al. (1987) Transurethral ultrasonic ureterolithotripsy using a solid-wire probe. Urology 29:531–532
30. Chausy C, Schmiedt E, Jocham D, et al. (1982) First clinical experience with extra corporeally induced destruction of kidney stones by shock waves. J Urol 127:417–420
31. Mobley TB, Myers DA, Grine WB, et al. (1993) Low-energy lithotripsy with the lithostar: treatment results with 19962 renal and ureteral calculi. J Urol 149:1419–1424
32. Bierkens AF, Hendrix AJ, deKort VJ, et al. (1992) Efficacy of second generation lithotriptors: a multicenter comparative study of 2206 extracorporeal shock wave lithotripsy treatments with the Siemens Lithostar, Dornier HM4, Wolf Piezolith 2300, Direx Tripter X-1 and Breakstone Lithotriptors. J Urol 148:1052–1056
33. Grasso M, Loisides P, Beaghler M, Bagley D (1995) The case for primary endoscopic management of upper urinary tract calculi. I. A critical review of 121 extracorporeal shock-wave lithotripsy failures. Urology 45:363–371
34. Segura JW, Preminger GM, Assimos DG, et al. (1994) Nephrolithiasis clinical guidelines panel summary report on the management of staghorn calculi. American Urological Association Nephrolithiasis Clinical Guidelines Panel. J Urol 151:1648–1651
35. Segura JW, Preminger GM, Assimos DG, et al. (1997) Ureteral stones clinical guidelines panel summary report on the management of ureteral calculi. J Urol 158:1915–1921
36. Bierkens AF, Hendrikx AJ, De La Rosette JJ, et al. (1998) Treatment of mid- and lower ureteric calculi: extracorporeal shock-wave lithotripsy vs. laser ureteroscopy. A comparison of costs, morbidity and effectiveness. Br J Urol 81:31–35

Calyceal Calculi

JOHN KOURAMBAS and GLENN M. PREMINGER

Summary. Since the advent of the "minimally invasive" era of urological surgery, there has been a progressive shift away from open renal surgery for stone disease. Open nephrolithotomy and pyelolithotomy have been all but replaced by percutaneous nephrolithotomy, ureteroscopy, shockwave lithotripsy, and laparoscopic approaches. With regards to calyceal calculi, shockwave lithotripsy (SWL) has rapidly become the treatment of choice. However, in some circumstances, percutaneous, ureteroscopic, laparoscopic, or even open operative approaches may be preferable. This chapter describes the current general treatment options available for calyceal calculi, and discusses treatment options for the management of specific troublesome calyceal stone scenarios.

Key Words. Calyceal calculi, Lithotripsy, Ureteroscopy, Percutaneous nephrolithotripsy

Pelvicalyceal Anatomy

When performing any endourological procedure, it is vital to understand the anatomy of the pelvicalyceal system completely. Failure to comprehend subtle anatomical factors may lead to treatment failures and complications that should otherwise have been avoided. Many urologists have difficulty interpreting the three-dimensional aspects of the calyceal system from the two-dimensional images of an intravenous pyelogram (IVP) or computerized tomogram (CT), which makes definitive localization of calyceal calculi difficult. Several studies have been performed that demonstrate the relationships of the calyceal system to the renal parenchyma and blood supply, which, in turn, facilitates the interpretation of radiographic studies and thus the performance of endourological procedures.

Comprehensive Kidney Stone Center, Division of Urology, Department of Surgery, Box 3167, Room 305, Baker House, Duke University Medical Center, Durham, NC 27710, USA

The normal kidney has between 4 and 12 (most often 8) calyces [1]. The upper and lower pole calyces are generally compound and lie at a variety of angles within the frontal plane of the kidney. The superior pole calyces are normally drained by a single infundibulum, while the lower pole system is more likely to have two distinct drainage systems [2]. The calyces may also be directed anteriorly or posteriorly. Standard current teaching suggests that the anterior calyces correspond to those that are more peripheral and lateral, as seen on an IVP, but some controversy still exists regarding this interpretation.

In 1901, Brodel [3] studied the internal anatomy of the kidneys, including the orientation of the calyces, and suggested that the anterior calyces were directed more medially than the posterior ones. However, more recently, Hodson [4] demonstrated that the mirror image of what Brodel described was, in actuality, the "true" calyceal orientation. These contradictory reports both examined ex vivo internal arrangements of the calyces. Kaye and Reinke [5] sought to study the calyceal relationships in vivo using CT imaging in order to provide clinically useful information for improved interpretation of the IVP and endourological procedures. This study found that the right kidneys tended to follow the pattern described by Brodel, while the left kidneys resembled the orientation that Hodson described. They also examined the relation of kidneys to the lateral aspect of the body and found that in 75% of kidneys (both left and right), the anterior calyces were positioned more laterally. Kidneys with posterior calyces that were laterally oriented were generally located on the right side. Finally, they concluded that in 74% of IVPs, the anterior calyces lie more laterally than the posterior calyces (65% of right kidneys and 83% of left kidneys).

As part of their analysis, Kaye and Reinke [5] also studied the orientation of the calyceal system in relation to the frontal plane of the kidney, as it would be viewed on a kidneys, ureter, bladder (KUB) or during fluoroscopy. The main aim of this study was to provide guidance for the proper placement of percutaneous access to the collecting system. They found that the posterior calyces of right kidneys averaged a 27° projection from the frontal plane, and that left kidneys averaged a 47° projection. If percutaneous access is desired on the right side with the patient in the prone position, rotating the patient right side up will project the posterior row of calyces nearly vertical, thus facilitating access. Since the posterior calyces on the left normally project further from the frontal plane, the patient need only be rotated approximately 10° upward to orient the calyces vertically.

A thorough understanding of the relationship of the internal vascular supply of the kidney with respect to the calyceal system should decrease the likelihood of a major vascular complication during endourological procedures, in particular percutaneous and laparoscopic surgery [6, 7]. Brodel [3] first described the lack of anastomoses between segmental arteries, while Graves [8] showed that there is a relatively constant pattern of arterial distribution that divides the kidney into specific anatomical segments. Sampaio [7] studied the relationship of these segmental arteries to the calyceal system using latex endocasts of 82 normal kidneys. Their study showed that in nearly 87% of kidneys, the arterial supply associated with the superior pole calyceal system consists of two arteries, one arising from the anterior division and one from the posterior division of the main renal artery. These arteries course anteriorly and posteriorly, but do not encircle an entire calyx. Thus, when performing endoscopic procedures, one should be aware of this relationship to avoid significant bleeding.

The artery to the interpolar calyces arises from the anterior division of the renal artery and demonstrates highly variable distribution patterns [7]. In the majority of cases, the arterial supply to the lower pole arises from the anterior division of the renal artery and courses anterior to the ureteropelvic junction or the lower pole infundibulum [7, 8]. The posterior arterial branch courses laterally and posteriorly immediately dorsal to the upper pole infundibulum or the more cephalad portion of the renal pelvis in an equal number of cases [7].

With regards to shockwave lithotripsy (SWL) and ureteroscopic approaches, knowledge of planar calyceal orientation and vascular anatomy is less vital. Here, calyceal relationships to the infundibulae and renal pelvis become most important [9, 10]. In particular, the lower pole calyceal anatomy strongly influences the outcome of SWL and ureteroscopic approaches for dependent lower pole stones. Anatomical studies have demonstrated three major features of the lower pole calyx that significantly influence post-SWL stone fragment clearance and ureteroscopic accessibility: infundibulopelvic angle, infundibular length, and infundibular width [11, 12].

Natural History of Calyceal Calculi

Prior to the advent of minimally invasive techniques to treat renal stone disease, many urologists were hesitant to remove calyceal stones that were discovered incidentally and were asymptomatic. Symptomatic calculi were treated by open surgery with relatively high morbidity compared with today's standards. In order to ascertain the optimal timing for surgical intervention for calyceal calculi, a recent study performed a retrospective analysis of 63 patients with 80 calyceal stones followed from diagnosis to passage of the stone, intervention, or censorship (defined as a "stone period") over an average of 7.4 years [13]. The majority of stones in these patients were located in lower pole calyces (70%), with 15% in the upper calyces and 7.5% in the mid-calyces. Of the 80 stones overall, 6% were dissolved with alkaline therapy (uric acid calculi), 16% passed spontaneously, 40% required open surgical intervention for removal, and 38% remained in situ at censorship. The indications for surgery were pain, recurrent infections, and hematuria. During the observation period, 45% of the stones increased in size, 68% of patients experienced symptoms of infection, and 51% experienced pain.

The investigators further subdivided the patients into three groups according to the duration of the "stone period" (2, 5, or 10 years), in order to make a better evaluation of the natural progression of their stone disease. Spontaneous stone passage decreased with increasing observation periods from 29% at 2 years to 13% at 5 years. None of the patients followed after 5 years spontaneously passed their stones. Symptoms of infection increased during the time period from 58% at 2 years to 83% at 10 years. A remarkable finding was that only 11% of the patients remained free of symptoms after 10 years of observation. In their analysis of the conservatively treated patients, 21% of the 5-year group and 38% of the 10-year group should have had surgery to avoid complications from their calyceal calculi. Of the 32 patients who eventually underwent surgery, the investigators believed that only 11 were performed at the appropriate time, since the other 23 patients had already experienced significant complications prior to surgery, including six patients who required nephrectomy for nonfunctioning kidneys or major stone mass.

Finally, the findings suggested that 80% of calyceal stones will require surgical intervention within 5 years following diagnosis, and that after 5 years, spontaneous stone passage is unlikely. The study recommends that with shockwave lithotripsy and percutaneous surgery readily available, when an indication for stone removal arises, intervention should be performed to prevent major complications secondary to stone disease. Moreover, patients who remain asymptomatic require close observation to detect any latent pathological changes. Nowadays, with the advent of improved ureteroscopic techniques, flexible ureteroscopy offers another alternative for the management of calyceal calculi in unique situations.

Management of Calyceal Calculi

The ultimate aim of treating any calculus is to render the patient not only symptom-free, but also stone-free, while preserving maximum renal function. The choice of an appropriate treatment strategy for calyceal calculi depends upon a number of distinct factors. Most important of these are stone size, location, and composition, as well as the anatomy of the urinary tract and the patient's overall medical condition.

Shockwave Lithotripsy

Since its introduction into clinical practice in 1980, shockwave lithotripsy has rapidly become the treatment of choice for calyceal calculi that are less than 2 cm in diameter [14–20]. This technology has allowed the treatment of over 95% of calyceal calculi, with minimal morbidity and complication rates of less than 5% [21, 22]. Using a variety of lithotriptors, many investigators have reported stone-free rates for these smaller calyceal calculi ranging between 48% and 98% [14, 16–18, 21, 23–27]. For any given location within the calyceal system, stone-free rates vary inversely with increasing stone size. Several studies have demonstrated that calyceal calculi less than 10 mm in greatest diameter will be associated with up to a 20% greater stone-free rate than corresponding calculi greater than 10 mm in diameter [16, 24]. Lingeman et al. [27] have demonstrated that the frequency of multiple treatments increases from 10% to 33% when treating stones sized 1–2 cm and 2–3 cm, respectively. Another report stated that nearly five SWL treatment sessions were required to achieve a successful outcome in calculi greater than 2.5 cm [24]. Current recommendations are that SWL monotherapy should be reserved for calyceal calculi less than 1.5–2.0 cm in diameter.

Complications following SWL appear to be directly correlated to increasing stone burden [21–23]. The incidence of steinstrasse (ureteral obstruction secondary to stone fragments within the ureter) is low following the treatment of calculi less than 10 mm diameter. However, the incidence of steinstrasse increases dramatically with increasing stone burden, and is up to 75% for some staghorn calculi [28]. The need for intervention because of obstruction has been reported to vary between 6% and 12% depending directly upon stone size [29, 30]. The use of preoperative ureteral stenting for larger calculi remains controversial. Although some investigators believe that stenting helps prevent obstruction and facilitates the passage of fragments, others have demonstrated that stents will only increase patient symptoms and will not reduce stone-related complications [31–35]. Ureteral stents may be indicated in patients with solitary kidneys, or where there is an unusual renal anatomy. The treatment of radiolucent or very small calculi may also benefit from prestenting in order to aid stone visualization.

Considering stones of similar composition, stone-free rates following SWL are not solely dependent upon the size of the calculi, but rather on size together with stone location. Stone-free rates are generally the highest for upper and mid-calyceal calculi, and significantly lower for lower calyceal stones. For upper and mid-calyceal calculi, one should expect stone-free rates in the range 70% to 90%, while those located in the lower calyces range between 50% and 70% [11, 16–18, 21–27, 36–38]. The presence of residual fragments following SWL, necessitating multiple or adjunct procedures, are also more commonly found not only in association with larger stones, but also for lower pole calyceal calculi [23, 27].

Many theories have been postulated as to the reason for the low rates of lower pole stone clearance after SWL. Elbahnasy et al. [11, 12] showed that the infundibulopelvic angle, the infundibular length, and the infundibular width are all vital factors that influence SWL success.

Most calculi are effectively fragmented with shockwave therapy. Exceptions to this finding primarily include some cystine stones and calcium oxalate monohydrate calculi [39]. Reduced fragmention may be secondary to the uniform structure and organic composition of these calculi, which may not vary greatly from the surrounding tissues [39, 40]. In addition, homogeneity of stone composition may also limit fragmentation. The energy transmitted to the stone at the tissue–stone interface and within the stone may not be sufficient to overcome the bonds that hold the stone together. In addition, when fragmentation of cystine stones does occur, the particle sizes tend to be much larger than those of other stones, and may lead to ureteral obstruction. It has been shown that cystine calculi less than 1 cm diameter can be treated effectively with SWL, but preoperative stenting is recommended [25]. A comparative study of SWL stone fragility demonstrated a progressive decrease in fragility from struvite, calcium apatite, uric acid, calcium oxalate dihydrate, and calcium oxalate monohydrate, to cystine [41]. Harder stones will usually require greater numbers of shocks than more fragile stones for complete fragmentation. Moreover, harder stones are more prone to other complications [42]. Approximately 2% of renal calculi will be refractory to adequate fragmentation with SWL and will require alternative forms of management [43].

Percutaneous Nephrolithotomy

Although SWL is the least invasive and most commonly used modality for treatment of calyceal calculi, there are many indications where percutaneous stone removal is preferred. Some of these indications include stone size, stone composition, aberrant renal anatomy, failure of SWL, and body habitus [43]. Percutaneous nephrolithotomy (PNL) is more invasive than SWL. However, to achieve the ultimate goal of a stone-free state, this technique often offers the best treatment option. Stone-free rates of up to 98% have been reported with PNL management of symptomatic calyceal stones [44, 45]. A particular common scenario where the percutaneous approach has significant advantages is that of the dependent lower pole calyceal calculus. As mentioned above, stone-free rates up to 50% less with SWL than with PNL may be expected [11, 12].

A study directly comparing lower pole calyceal calculi treated with SWL or PNL found that with stone size over 2–3 cm, stone-free rates using percutaneous treatments were nearly 50% greater than those obtained by SWL (90% vs. 43%) [27]. In addition, the requirements for multiple procedures are significantly higher in patients treated with SWL. Very large or hard calyceal calculi may require multiple percutaneous procedures to render the patient free of stones. Some of these patients may benefit from combined PNL and SWL. Percutaneous nephrolithotomy is generally performed first, followed by SWL of inaccessible residual stones. If large or multiple fragments remain, then a second percutaneous procedure can readily be performed through the preexisting nephrostomy tract.

Hard calyceal calculi (such as calcium oxalate monohydrate or cystine) are ideally treated with PNL, especially when the stone size is greater than 1.5 cm. Direct visual fragmentation and stone removal allow for significantly better stone-free rates than SWL monotherapy.

SWL is also unlikely to be an effective treatment in those patients with some form of anatomical restriction to normal urinary drainage, with reported failure rates of 70%. Percutaneous procedures are most effective in the management of calculi in these patients, since both stones and the anatomical defect may be treated concurrently.

Ureteropelvic junction (UPJ) obstruction, infundibular stenosis, and calyceal diverticulae are specific examples of conditions that impede urinary flow and passage of stone fragments. In addition, some patients may have an obvious stone-filled calyx which is likely to be an infection stone (as determined by the clinical presentation of fever and/or recurrent infections). If this calyx fails to visualize on an intravenous urogram, SWL should be avoided [46]. This picture may represent an obstructed pyocalyx, and attempts at SWL may result in sepsis. The treatment of choice for these patients is percutaneous stone extraction and drainage of the infected system [46].

Percutaneous procedures should also be considered when other treatment modalities have failed to treat the calyceal stone sufficiently. Incomplete stone removal most commonly occurs following SWL as the stone may not adequately fragment, multiple large fragments may remain despite several treatments, or obstruction of the system may prevent adequate passage of fragments.

It is only in extremely rare circumstances that percutaneous procedures cannot be performed. These situations may occur when percutaneous access cannot be obtained. Many urologists and radiologists are wary of attempting percutaneous access into the superior calyces because of the increased risk of violating the pleural space, with subsequent pneumothorax, hydrothorax, or hemothorax formation. These complications occur in 1.6% to 3% of patients undergoing supra-12th rib access [6, 21, 47]. For supra-11th rib (and higher) access, intrathoracic complications occur in up to 25% of patients [47]. However, all of these complications, when appropriately recognized, are easily managed with minimal intervention or patient morbidity. Thus, supracostal approaches should not be avoided, since with complex calyceal stones they often offer the only viable treatment option that can render the patient stone-free. One reported method describes a renal displacement technique which allows for percutaneous access to the superior calyces with decreased intrathoracic morbidity [48]. This technique employs percutaneous placement of a firm sheath through a lower or central calyx, which can then be used to torque to a kidney caudally, thus bringing the superior calyx below the 12 rib. However, this technique may result in renal lacerations and significant blood loss, complications not easily recognizable or manageable. Therefore, we do not perform this maneuver.

Ureterorenoscopy

Although SWL and PNL are still the mainstays in treating renal calyceal calculi, ureterorenoscopic techniques now offer an alternative treatment modality. With recent improvements in flexible ureteroscopes, fiberoptic and imaging technologies, enhanced stone fragmentation, and retrieval devices, flexible ureterorenoscopy offers not only a viable, but in certain circumstances a preferable, management modality for symptomatic calyceal calculi. With the use of actively deflectable ureteroscopes, all the calyces may be accessed in over 95% of kidneys, including lower pole calyces [49].

The first truly flexible intracorporeal lithotripsy device, electrohydraulic lithotripsy (EHL), advanced flexible ureteroscopy from a purely diagnostic tool to a therapeutic maneuver. However, the explosive nature of EHL fragmenation often results in damage to the collecting system or the ureteroscope. The introduction of the holmium laser, and in particular the 200-μm holmium laser fiber,

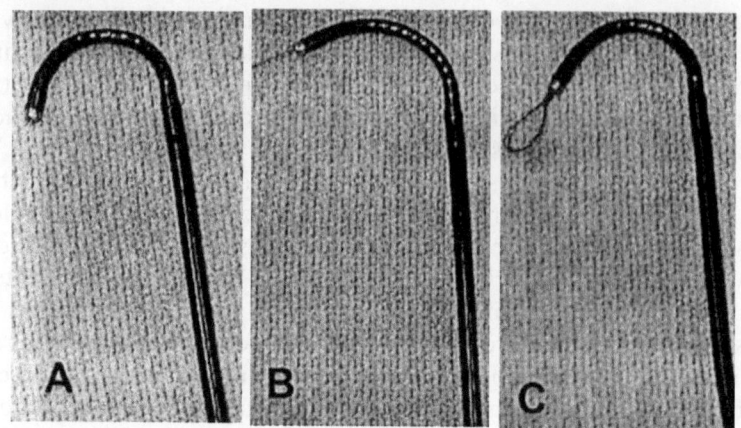

FIG. 1. 7.5-F flexible ureterorenoscope at: **A** full deflection; **B** with 200μ holmium laser fiber; **C** with 3.2-F nitinol basket

has revolutionized ureterorenoscopic lithotripsy. As the maximal ureteroscopic deflectability is compromised by only 7% to 16% when the 200-μm fiber is passed through the ureteroscope, most calyceal stones can be fragmented in situ (Fig. 1) [50].

In some situations where a calyceal calculus cannot be fragmented in situ owing to loss of deflection (secondary to the passage of the laser fiber), small nitinol baskets or graspers can be used to manipulate the stone into a less dependent calyx for fragmentation (Fig. 1) [51, 52]. This technique has allowed complete access to calculi located anywhere in the intrarenal collecting system, with a subsequent increase in stone-free rates. Early reports described only a 50% success rate in treating renal and calyceal calculi ureteroscopically, but more recent studies have demonstrated successful treatments in over 80% of patients [51, 53–57].

There have been other reports of patients with radiolucent, calyceal calculi that can be effectively treated with flexible ureteroscopy [56]. In addition, ureteroscopic stone fragmentation or extraction is an excellent option in patients with bleeding diatheses where SWL and percutaneous procedures may be contraindicated [56, 58].

Most recently, a flexible pneumatic lithotripsy (lithoclast) probe has become available for use with flexible ureteroscopes. The excellent fragmentation ability and safety of pneumatic lithotripsy has been well documented [59, 60]. With the introduction of the flexible lithoclast probe, renal calculi can now be treated with increased efficacy, in particular upper and mid-pole calyceal stones. However, in vitro studies have documented decreased fragmentation capabilities with increased deflection of the flexible lithoclast probe (Fig. 2) [61]. Taking all these factors into account, the holmium laser remains the intracorporeal lithotripsy device of choice for ureteroscopic management of calyceal stones.

FIG. 2. 7.5-F flexible ureterorenoscope with
0.5-mm flexible lithoclast probe

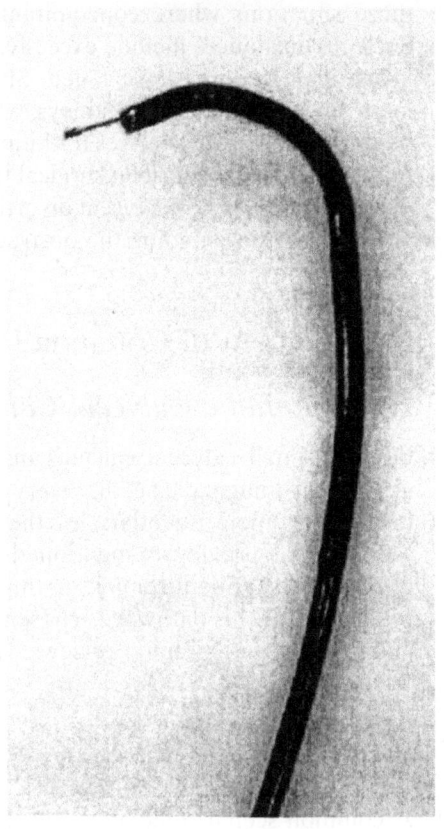

Laparoscopic Surgery

Recently, laparoscopic surgery has emerged as a viable treatment option for
patients with various renal disorders. Laparoscopic nephrectomy is still considered an advanced laparoscopic procedure, but may be performed as an alternative to simple open nephrectomy [62]. If the kidney is chronically infected,
significant scarring and adhesions may make laparoscopic procedures even more
technically challenging. A recent report describes the use of laparoscopic partial
nephrectomy for the management of calyceal stone disease [63]. Other reported
laparoscopic procedures for calyceal stone disease include laparoscopic pyelo
and nephrolithotomies [64–66]. However, all of these procedures are technically
challenging, and should only be performed by those with extensive laparoscopic
experience.

Open Surgery

Although open renal stone surgery is now rarely performed, nephrolithotomy
remains a viable option in the treatment of large calyceal calculi, especially in

those situations where concomitant reconstructive procedures are warranted. Such circumstances include excessive calyceal stone burden, or where minimally invasive procedures have failed. Simple nephrectomy is an appropriate treatment for nonfunctioning kidneys, while anatrophic nephrolithotomy and radial nephrotomy are alternatives for kidneys with adequate function. Partial nephrectomy offers a form of open surgical treatment for calyceal calculi associated with obstructed calyces or calyceal diverticula, where there is limited functional renal parenchyma surrounding the obstructed calyx [67].

Management of Common Problematic Scenarios

Asymptomatic Calyceal Calculi

Often, a small calyceal calculus may be incidentally identified during routine abdominal imaging. The discovery of an asymptomatic calculus often results in a management quandary for the urologist and undue stress for the patient. Although, as previously mentioned, a completely stone-free status is desirable, as long as the patient remains asymptomatic, a conservative approach is entirely reasonable. If this pathway is chosen, we recommend a full metabolic evaluation and regular radiographic reviews. However, if symptoms arise, intervention is warranted.

Small Nonobstructing Symptomatic Calyceal Calculi

A common scenario facing the urologist is the patient with small, nonobstructing, calyceal calculi. As mentioned above, in the majority of these situations the stones are asymptomatic, and observation is usually recommended. However, when these patients complain of flank or abdominal discomfort or are found to have microscopic hematuria, it becomes unclear whether the stone is the source of the problem.

In the past, several reports have shown that surgical treatment of such stones can relieve pain in the majority of cases [68, 69]. These stones can now be managed less invasively with SWL. Yet, with several lithotriptors, the visualization of small calculi may be extremely difficult, especially when fluoroscopy is used. In this situation, a preoperatively placed ureteral catheter will allow the injection of contrast, with adequate visualization of the involved calyx. Several reports have described the successful treatment of small calyceal stones with SWL [70, 71]. Over 90% of patients have achieved complete or significant pain relief following SWL treatment.

Another viable treatment option for small symptomatic calyceal calculi is ureteroscopic fragmentation. Stone-free rates of up to 90% have been reported for small calyceal calculi treated in this manner [57]. We currently offer patients with small, questionably symptomatic calyceal stones either SWL or ureteroscopic treatment only if conservative measures have failed. However, we strongly impress upon the patient that the stone may not be the cause of their discomfort, and that their pain may not resolve following the intervention.

Lower Pole Calyceal Calculi

As previously outlined, knowledge of the anatomy of the collecting system in relation to a lower pole calyceal calculus is vital when assessing potential treatment options and outcomes. Although SWL is the treatment of choice for approximately 90% of calyceal calculi, almost all the literature describes a lower stone-free rate for lower calyceal stones compared with those in mid- and superior pole calyces [17, 18, 24, 26, 38, 44, 72]. Some studies have reported stone-free rates (post-SWL) as high as 79%, but most series have shown significantly poorer stone-free rates of generally between 40% and 58% [11, 17, 37, 38]. With this low stone-free rate, alternative procedures may be warranted to improve the overall outcomes of lower pole stone management.

One would suspect that if the decreased clearance of stone fragments following SWL is solely dependent on gravity, such maneuvers as simple inversion therapy would significantly increase stone-free rates. However, reports in the literature are conflicting, suggesting that gravity alone is not responsible for the poor results [73, 74]. In fact, one study where the patients were treated with inversion therapy actually had a lower rate of stone clearance compared with controls (65% vs. 84%) [73]. While controlled inversion therapy has not been proved to facilitate the passage of lower pole fragments following SWL, other investigators have attempted different maneuvers to promote their passage [75, 76]. One group reported an improved stone-free rate from 54% to 71% at 3 months follow-up using a cystoscopically placed cobra catheter to irrigate the lower pole calyx during SWL [75]. However, with many current SWL treatments being performed under limited analgesia, the routine placement of a cobra catheter would significantly increase the morbidity and costs of SWL. While this adjunctive procedure did not add significant morbidity to the treatment, long-term studies should be performed to determine the overall efficacy of irrigation techniques.

Sampaio and Aragao [9] have performed rather elegant anatomical studies of the lower pole calyceal system in order to determine the possible causes of decreased clearance of stone fragments from this area. They discovered that 57% of lower pole systems are drained by multiple calyces, and theorized that this anatomical feature drains more poorly than those systems with only one midline calyceal infundibulum receiving fused calyces. Another important anatomical feature promoting decreased drainage was believed to be related to the angle between the renal pelvis and the lower pole infundibulum. If this angle was less than 90° (which occurred in 26% of the kidneys studied), drainage would be impaired, and fewer fragments would pass. Other investigators have also studied the impact of lower pole anatomy on SWL success. Elbahnassy et al. [11, 12] demonstrated that when the infundibulopelvic angle is large (>70°), or the infundibulum is long (>3 cm), or the infundibulum is narrow (<3 mm), the SWL stone-free rate is significantly decreased as stone fragment clearance is hampered. In fact, when all three factors coexisted, they report a stone-free rate of less than 50%.

As with calculi in other calyces, stone-free rates for SWL treatment of lower calyceal calculi vary significantly with stone size. These rates ranged from 60% to 78% and from 25% to 50% for stones less than 1 cm diameter and stones greater than 2 cm diameter, respectively [24, 38, 44, 72]. In comparison, percutaneous treatment of lower pole stones ranging in diameter from 4 mm to 27 mm yielded stone-free rates of 85% in one investigation. Others have shown a stone-free rate of up to 90% [44, 45]. A recently metaanalysis compared the results of SWL and PNL for lower calyceal calculi [44]. The overall stone-free rate of SWL was 60%, while that for PNL was 90%. When stratifying treatments according to stone size, it appeared that for stones less than 1 cm diameter, the stone-free rates were 74% for SWL and 100% for PNL. For larger stones (greater than 2 cm), the stone-free rate for SWL decreased to 33% while that for PNL was 94%. From these data, one may conclude that PNL may be the most appropriate treatment for lower calyceal calculi, especially for stones larger than 1 cm. However, this is with the added risk of complications, increased hospital stay, and significantly increased cost.

A recently available alternative to SWL and PNL in the management of lower calyceal stones is flexible holmium laser ureterorenoscopic lithotripsy. This technique is especially useful in situations where SWL and PNL would result in increased morbidity or would be technically difficult to perform. We have used this approach in patients with lower pole calculi for whom previous SWL has failed, who have a bleeding diathesis, who are morbidly obese (precluding SWL for weight restriction reasons and PNL for technical access reasons), or who have hard stones such as calcium oxalate monohydrate or cystine (which are generally resistant to SWL) [51, 77].

To preserve maximal ureteroscopic deflectability, we routinely use a 200-μm holmium laser fiber. However, when entry into the lower pole is precluded by loss of deflection caused by the passage of the laser fiber, we have found the use of flexible nickel–titanium (nitinol) stone-retrieval devices indispensable. In particular, we have used the 3.2 F tipless nitinol basket (Cook Urological, Spencer, IN, USA) and the 2.6 F nitinol grasper (Microvasive/Boston Scientific, Natick, MA, USA). These allow the stone to be displaced into a mid- or upper (preferably) calyx, and thus allow for easier access and fragmentation with the less-deflected holmium laser fiber. The 2.6 F grasper, in particular, is our device of choice, because it allows for increased irrigation (and thus optical vision), and less morbidity because stone disengagement is more easily accomplished than with a basket (Fig. 3). Using this technique (Fig. 4), we have been able to fragment 100% of lower calyceal stones and achieve a stone-free rate of 85% [51].

Calyceal Diverticular Calculi

Calyceal diverticula are urine-filled cavities connected to the normal collecting system by a narrow isthmus. The cavity is lined with nonsecretory transitional

FIG. 3. 2.6-F nitinol grasper

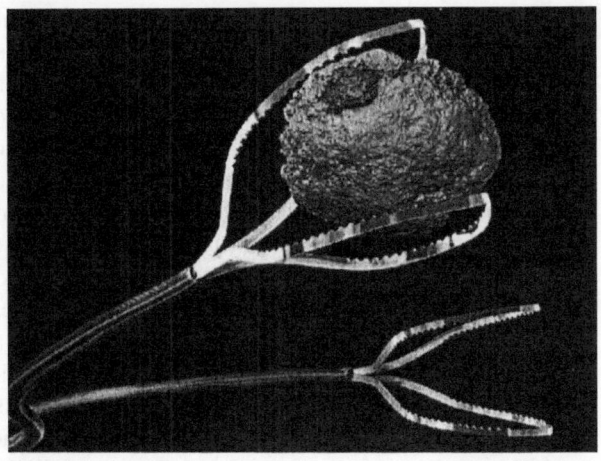

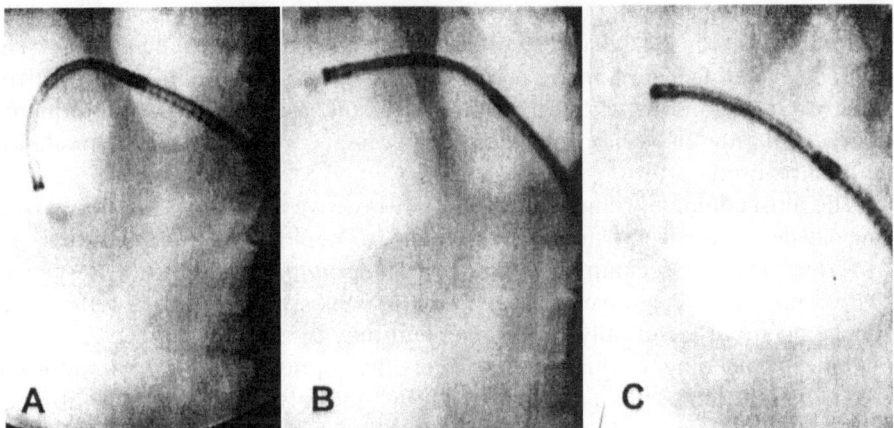

FIG. 4. **A** Ureterorenoscope in lower pole calyx. **B** Calculus repositioned into mid-calyx.
C Calculus after holmium laser fragmentation

epithelium and fills with urine in a retrograde fashion. These diverticula are generally detected incidentally on routine IVP, and have an incidence of less than 1% [78]. The exact etiology of these anomalies is controversial, although most agree that they are likely congenital, since the incidence is nearly identical in children and adults. While most calyceal diverticula remain asymptomatic, flank pain, hematuria, and/or recurrent infection may be the presenting symptom(s). The incidence of calculi within calyceal diverticula has been reported to be between 10% and 50% [79]. These calculi often cause a localized inflammatory reaction which can lead to fibrosis of the diverticular wall and possible stenosis or obliteration of the connecting isthmus [80]. Such stones occasionally pass spontaneously, but require intervention if they become symptomatic. The most common indication for treatment of calyceal diverticular calculi is ipsilateral flank pain; others include recurrent infection or persistent gross hematuria.

Treatment options for calculi within calyceal diverticula are numerous, ranging from open surgery to SWL. Most investigators agree, however, that eradication of the diverticulum should accompany attempts to render the patient free of stones, in order to prevent subsequent stone formation or other complications associated with the diverticulum. Many investigators have attempted to manage diverticular stones with SWL, but with varying results. The reported stone-free rates for calyceal diverticular calculi treated exclusively with SWL range between 4% and 58% [81–85]. Fragmentation of the stone is often successful in these instances, but the narrow neck of the diverticulum and the limited flow of urine hinder the passage of the stone fragments. A significantly higher stone-free rate (58%) may be achieved by treating selected patients with small calculi (less than 1.5 cm) and a radiographically patent diverticular neck [84].

Although stone-free rates in these series of SWL for stones in calyceal diverticula are generally low, between 70% and 80% of the patients treated in this manner reported resolution of their symptoms [81–85]. It appears that SWL monotherapy for calculi in calyceal diverticula may be beneficial in selected patients, yielding symptomatic relief. However, in those patients with recurrent pain or infections, in whom a stone-free result is important, or in situations where ablation of the diverticulum is necessary, other treatment modalities should be used.

The most commonly employed minimally invasive alternative to SWL in treating calyceal diverticular stones is percutaneous nephrolithotomy. A direct puncture into the diverticulum under radiographic guidance is possible, especially with a posterior-lying diverticulum. Percutaneous approaches to anterior diverticula are more technically challenging and may cause parenchymal damage or significant bleeding. In this circumstance, other options may be more appropriate. If a guide wire cannot pass easily through the calyceal neck, a bent-tipped or cobra catheter may help direct the wire. Alternatively, the wire can be coiled within the diverticulum and the nephrostomy tract dilated to allow access to the cavity.

Recently, we have reviewed our series of percutaneous management for calyceal diverticular stones where a "neoinfundibulotomy" was created (when passage of the wire through the diverticular infundibulum was not possible). In these cases, we puncture directly into the main collecting system, traversing the diverticulum en route. Dilation is then performed over the guide wire, thus creating a new communication between the diverticulum and the main renal collecting system, a "neoinfundibulum" (Fig. 5). All patients treated in this manner were rendered symptom-free and stone-free; 75% of diverticula were completely absent at 3 months, and the remainder were significantly reduced in size.

The stone-free results of diverticular calculi treated using percutaneous techniques have been far superior to those treated with SWL alone. Most investigators report these stone-free rates to be greater than 80% [83, 85–87]. A recent

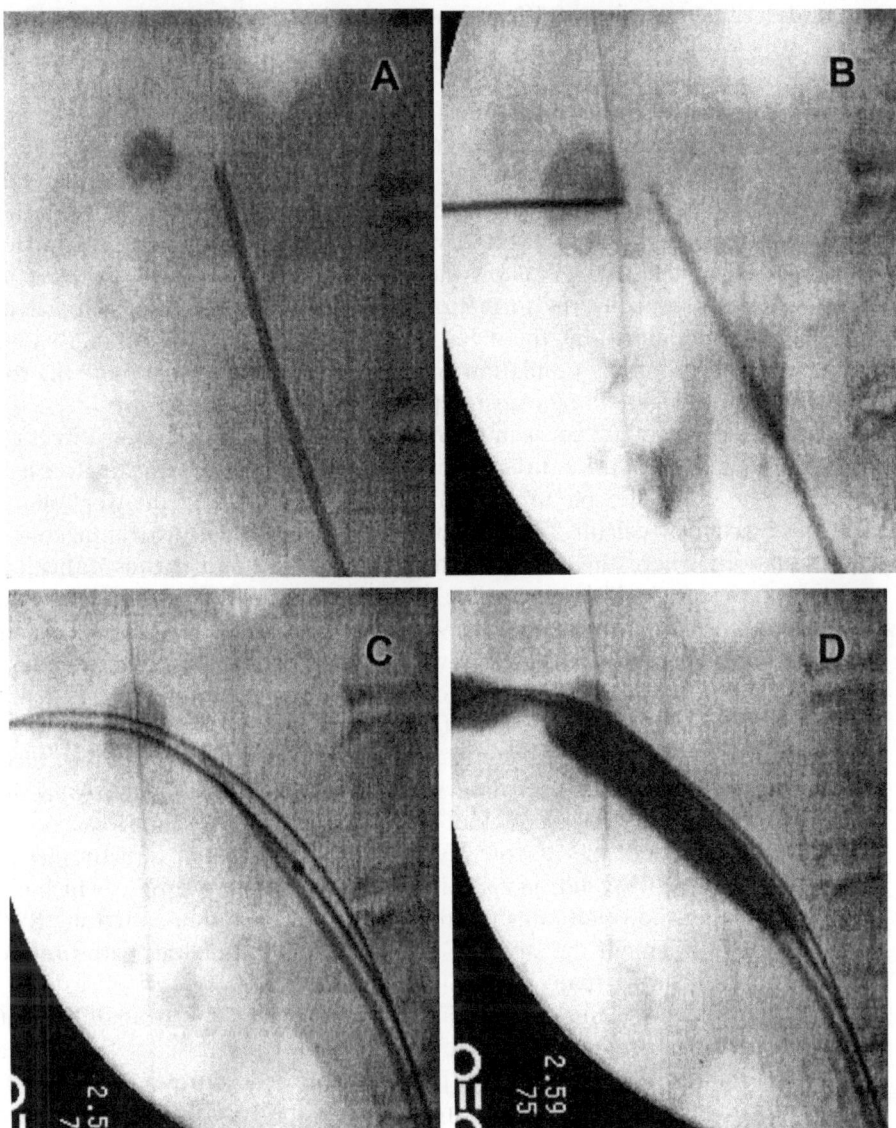

FIG. 5. **A** Stone in upper pole calyceal diverticulum. **B** Diverticulum punctured with access needle. **C** Wire through wall of diverticulum, into main collecting system, and down ureter. **D** Balloon dilation of "neo-infundibulum"

report described a series of 19 patients with diverticular calculi treated percutaneously, with 18 patients (95%) becoming stone-free [87]. Moreover, these studies indicate that more than 80% of patients can be expected to be rendered free of infections and other symptoms [83, 85–87].

Unlike SWL treatment, percutaneous measures allow for the management of the diverticulum itself. If a substantial amount of renal parenchyma overlies the diverticulum, the calyceal neck should be dilated, the cavity wall fulgurated, and the nephrostomy tube placed through the opening for a period of approximately 3–4 weeks. This maneuver will allow the neck to heal open, thereby preventing stenosis and, theoretically, the formation of new stones. When the parenchyma over the diverticulum is thin, the diverticular wall as well as the isthmus should be fulgurated to promote granulation and obliteration of the cavity, and the roof of the diverticulum should be resected [85].

Owing to the recent advances in fiberoptic technology, which allow direct retrograde visualization of the entire pelvicalyceal system, several investigators have advocated the use of flexible ureterorenoscopic techniques for the treatment of calyceal diverticular calculi. This technique may be especially advantageous in those situations where the diverticulum lies anteriorly, and is thus difficult to access percutaneously. Using a flexible ureterorenoscope, the diverticular neck may be visualized directly, and a guide wire passed through the infundibulum and into the diverticular cavity. Once the wire is coiled within the diverticulum, a dilating balloon may be placed over the wire. The calyceal isthmus may then be dilated to 15 F, thus allowing passage of the flexible ureteroscope into the diverticulum (Fig. 6). Once direct access to the diverticulum is obtained, the calculi within it may be fragmented using laser or electrohydraulic lithotripsy. An added advantage of the holmium laser is that the diverticular cavity lining can be fulgurated and, if needed, the narrow diverticular infundibulum directly incised. The fulguration usually results in a significant inflammatory response, which ultimately granulates and obliterates the diverticular space. Others advocate SWL pretreatment to fragment the stone to avoid potential difficulties with ureteroscopic techniques and virtually ensure fragmentation [88].

Stone-free rates using this ureterorenoscopic technique are around 70% [56, 88]. Other investigators have used ureteroscopically guided access to calyceal diverticula to improve the outcome of percutaneous procedures [89].

Following the conclusion of the ureterorenoscopic procedure, an internal ureteral stent should be placed across the dilated diverticular neck to ensure that the opening remains patent. Although this procedure is less invasive than percutaneous management, it may be technically challenging for those with limited experience of using flexible ureterorenoscopy.

More recently, laparoscopic techniques have been used to solve the problem of complex calyceal diverticular calculi [65, 66]. In two reports, the diverticula were located anteriorly and were exophytic. During the operative procedure, the roof of the diverticulum was resected, the neck obliterated, and the diverticular lining fulgurated. A laparoscopic, argon-beam coagulator can facilitate this process. An important step in this operation is the preoperative placement of

FIG. 6. Flexible ureterorenoscope in calyceal diverticulum over guide wire

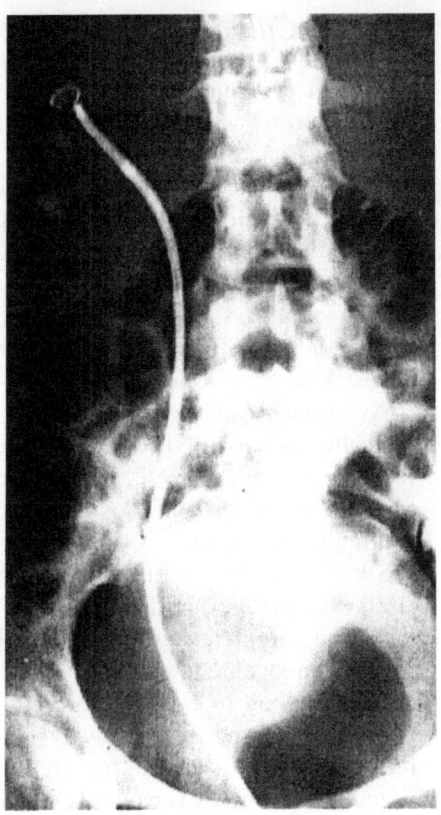

a ureteral catheter, through which methylene blue or indigo carmine can be
injected to detect leakage from the collecting system out through the ablated
diverticulum. If this connection remains patent, a fistula may occur. Both of the
patients in these reports did extremely well without any significant complications.
Laparoscopic procedures may provide an excellent alternative to open surgery
for the management of complex diverticular calculi, especially in the hands of
experienced laparoscopic surgeons.

   While minimally invasive techniques dominate current management of calculi
in calyceal diverticula, open surgical stone removal and diverticulectomy were
the mainstay of treatment for this condition in the past. Open surgical procedures
may still be the most appropriate form of therapy for some patients today, especially for those individuals where a stone-free state is essential. Various open procedures have been described for treatment of these calculi, including resection
of the diverticular roof with obliteration of the calyceal neck and lining, as well
as partial nephrectomy. Intraoperative sonography may facilitate the localization
of the calculi-containing diverticulum, particularly if a substantial amount of
parenchyma overlies the area.

Cystine Calyceal Calculi

Although cystinuria is rare, accounting for only 1%–2% of all adult urinary calculi, and 6%–8% of pediatric urinary calculi, cystinuric patients suffer from high recurrence rates and thus may require multiple treatments and interventions [90–94]. Recent advances in endourological techniques, coupled with more sophisticated metabolic management, has led to a significant overall improvement in the cystinuric patient's care. Unfortunately, medical management is often unsuccessful, with failure rates as high as 60%–70% being reported [95, 96]. Many patients require surgical intervention, often on a frequent basis [97]. Studies have reported that cystinuric patients suffer an average of 1.22 stone episodes per year during long-term follow-up [98].

As surgical intervention is often necessary, current treatment options are typically SWL or PNL, with open surgery being reserved for endourologically recalcitrant stones [99]. Until recently, small-caliber flexible ureteroscopes were not available, and thus the retrograde ureterorenoscopic approach was not routinely considered.

SWL is widely used for the management of smaller cystine stones (<15mm) [100]. Some reports advocate SWL for treating larger cystine stone burdens, including complete staghorn calculi [101]. However, the overall results of SWL for the management of cystine stones are generally suboptimal, with stone-free rates as low as 10% [102]. As cystine stones are often resistant to SWL, many cystinuric patients ultimately require percutaneous stone removal. Moreover, repeat PNL procedures for treatment of recurrent cystine stones is often required, and often repeatedly. While PNL has been demonstrated to be relatively safe and without long-term sequelae, in some instances scarring of the renal parenchyma can occur [103, 104]. Although PNL remains the management option of choice for cystine calyceal stones, with the need for repeat procedures, cumulative deleterious effects of this scarring are possible. Although the long-term sequelae of repeat PNL is not known, the associated perinephric fibrosis can make the frequently necessary repeat procedures exponentially more difficult.

Laser lithotripsy was initially thought to be ineffective in fragmenting cystine calculi, with pulsed-dye lasers having only a 10% fragmentation effect compared with its results with calcium oxalate calculi [105, 106]. However, with the advent of holmium laser lithotripsy, cystine stones can now be completely fragmented (Fig. 7). Holmium laser fragmentation studies of various stone compositions (utilizing constant energy and fiber sizes) have shown that cystine calculi fragment as easily as uric acid calculi and more easily than calcium oxalate monohydrate calculi. Our experience supports this finding, as do other studies of cystine stones [94, 107]. We reported on three cystinuric patients with a significant stone burden (mean 2.2 cm) who were treated with holmium laser lithotripsy via a 7.5-F flexible ureterorenoscope. Two of the three patients were rendered completely stone-free, with the third having only small (<3 mm), asymptomatic fragments at 3-month follow-up [77].

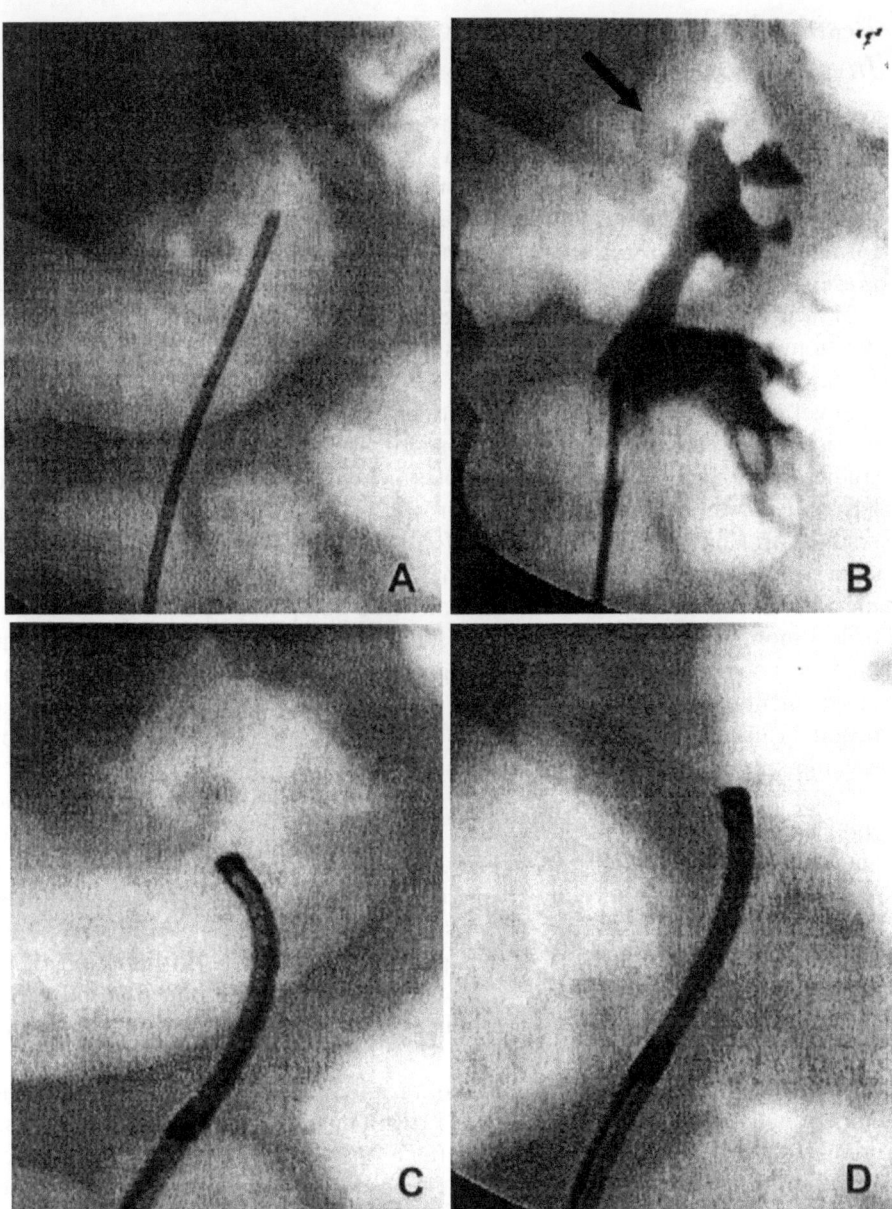

FIG. 7. Right upper pole calyceal cystine renal calculus. **A** Kidneys, ureter, bladder (KUB) with ureteral catheter in upper pole calyx. **B** Retrograde pyelogram demonstrating stone in medial upper pole location (*arrow*). **C** Flexible ureterorenoscope with holmium laser fiber in place. **D** Complete fragmentation of calculus

Residual Fragments Following Minimally Invasive Procedures

With the introduction of less invasive procedures for the management of nephrolithiasis, less emphasis has been placed on the significance of any remaining stone material. Small stone fragments (<5 mm) are considered by some to be "clinically insignificant." However, several studies have noted an increase in stone formation, growth of residual fragments, and/or symptomatic episodes with the presence of residual calculi following SWL [108–113]. A recent report noted a 71% probability of patients with "clinically insignificant" residual fragments developing symptoms, or requiring subsequent intervention, or both over a 5-year period following SWL [113].

Several investigators have reported their experience with early retreatment of persistent calyceal fragments following primary SWL [114, 115]. Both of these studies employed a piezoelectric lithotriptor which requires no anesthesia and has limited complications. One group prospectively retreated 25 patients who had residual fragments within 2 months following initial SWL and compared the stone-free rates with an untreated, control group [114]. They found that 40% of the retreated group were rendered stone-free compared with only 4% of controls 3 months after retreatment. The second report demonstrated that retreatment was only successful for stone fragments in normal calyces, while clearance of fragments was unlikely in dilated calyces [115]. Aggressive retreatment of residual calyceal calculi may therefore be indicated if anesthesia-free lithotripsy is commonly available.

Since residual fragments can act as a nidus for further stone formation, one should consider prophylactic medical therapy to prevent new stone formation and/or growth of residual stone fragments. After SWL, or any other modality of stone removal, the underlying physiological or metabolic defects for recurrent stone formation persist. Growth of existing stones and possible formation of new calculi may be inevitable because of supersaturation of stone-forming substances and/or the lack of stone-inhibitors. However, appropriate medical therapy initiated after fragmentation, with or without evidence of residual calculi, may control metabolically active stone disease.

Two recent studies support the role of prophylactic medical therapy following stone removal, especially when residual fragments are present [116, 117]. A randomized, prospective trial studied the effects of sodium citrate therapy or conservative measures (dietary limitation of dairy products and salty foods, and increased fluids) on residual fragments following shockwave lithotripsy [116]. There was a 75% reduction in the clearance of calcium stone fragments in those patients receiving sodium citrate. However, only 32% of the patients receiving conservative measures had clearance of their calcium stone fragments. Similarly, in patients with residual struvite fragments, nonselective medical therapy with sodium citrate cleared residual fragments in 86% of patients, whereas only 40% of patients receiving conservative measures had clearance of their struvite stone fragments.

The same study also looked at the effect of nonspecific sodium citrate therapy on stone growth and/or reaggregation of residual fragments. It was found that

47% of patients had growth of residual stones or reaggregation of stone fragments while having conservative treatment. In contrast, stone growth reaggregation was only noted in 5% of those patients receiving sodium citrate therapy. This study concluded that persistence and growth are common findings in the natural history of residual fragments following shockwave lithotripsy. Moreover, citrate therapy appears to increase fragment clearance rates and reduce the growth and agglomeration of residual stone fragments following shockwave lithotripsy.

Another study evaluated 80 patients who had all undergone a full metabolic evaluation following shockwave lithotripsy and who were given selective medical therapy [117]. However, only 60% remained on this therapy. This study examined the effectiveness of selective medical therapy on active stone formation during long-term follow-up. Specific attention was directed toward the significance of residual stone fragments and their effect on stone growth and/or recurrent stone formation. Two groups of stone-free patients (with and without continued medical therapy) and two groups of patients with residual fragments (with and without continued medical therapy) were studied. All patients were similar with respect to their demographic parameters, average age, time to follow-up, prelithotripsy number of stones, and postlithotripsy stone burden.

Patients with or without residual fragments who continued on specific medical therapy had a significant decrease in their stone formation rate. In stone-free patients, medical therapy after shockwave lithotripsy reduced recurrent stone formation by 91%. In patients with residual fragments after SWL, medical therapy produced an 81% reduction in the stone-formation rate. There were 31 patients who did not continue on specific medical therapy following lithotripsy. Over 77% of these patients were noted to have persistent metabolic stone activity, even though metabolic stone activity could be reduced to 36% with the administration of appropriate medical therapy. Moreover, of the patients with residual calculi who were managed with medical therapy, only 16% had active stone growth. Conversely, of the patients with residual calculi who were not managed with medical therapy, 54.5% demonstrated active stone growth.

These data suggest that residual stone fragments, following minimally invasive procedures for calyceal calculi, do pose a significant risk for stone growth and/or recurrent stone formation. Therefore, all attempts (within reason) to render a patient stone-free should be made. Aggressive metabolic management should also be instituted to avoid the inherent risks and possible complications of recurrent stone fragment growth. Continued patient compliance and appropriate physician follow-up is mandatory to ensure the effective prevention of metabolic stone activity.

Conclusions

Nowadays, our approach to managing calyceal calculi has been significantly altered owing to rapid changes and improvements in endoscopic and shockwave lithotripsy technology. Although these changes have virtually eliminated the need for open surgical stone removal, one must still maintain a clear understanding of the renal and collecting system anatomy in order to manage patients with calyceal stones safely and effectively. With the minimally invasive techniques available, one should consider treating even asymptomatic, incidentally detected, calyceal calculi, since the majority of these stones may eventually become symptomatic and/or require intervention. While most calyceal calculi can be managed effectively with shockwave lithotripsy, large, lower pole, and "SWL-resistant" stones may be more appropriately treated with either PNL or ureterorenoscopic techniques. Flexible ureterorenoscopy also offers further advantages as an excellent adjunct procedure for the removal of small, residual, calyceal stone fragments following SWL or PNL. Endoscopic approaches should also be considered for the management of common problematic calyceal calculi, such as lower pole stones, cystine stones, and calculi within a calyceal diverticulum. Although rarely performed, open surgical stone removal should be considered as a viable treatment option for calyceal calculi, especially when a large stone burden is present or when concomitant procedures are needed. Finally, one must remember that the mode of removal will have no effect on recurrent stone formation. Therefore, metabolic stone evaluation and appropriate medical therapy should be considered to prevent the growth of residual stone fragments, as well as to inhibit the formation of new calculi.

References

1. Kaye KW (1983) Renal anatomy for endourologic stone removal. J Urol 130:647–648
2. Sampaio FJB, Mandarim-de-Lacerda CA (1988) Anatomic classification of the kidney collecting system for endourologic procedures. J Endourol 2:247–251
3. Brodel M (1901) The intrinsic blood vessels of the kidney and their significance in nephrotomy. Bull Johns Hopkins Hosp 12:10
4. Hodson J (1972) The lobar structure of the kidney. Br J Urol 44:246
5. Kaye KW, Reinke DB (1984) Detailed caliceal anatomy for endourology. J Urol 132:1085–1088
6. Lee WJ, Smith AD, Cubelli V, Badlani GH, Lewin B, Vernace F, Cantos E (1987) Complications of percutaneous nephrolithotomy. Am J Roentgenol 148:177–180
7. Sampaio F (1992) Review: anatomic background for intrarenal endourologic surgery. J Endourol 6:301–304
8. Graves FT (1954) The anatomy of the intrarenal arteries and its application to segmental resection of the kidney. Br J Surg 42:132
9. Sampaio FJ, Aragao AH (1992) Inferior pole collecting system anatomy: its probable role in extracorporeal shock wave lithotripsy. J Urol 147:322–324
10. Sampaio FJ, Aragao AH (1994) Limitations of extracorporeal shockwave lithotripsy for lower caliceal stones: anatomic insight. J Endourol 8:241–247
11. Elbahnasy AM, Shalhav AL, Hoenig DM, Elashry OM, Smith DS, McDougall EM, Clayman RV (1998) Lower caliceal stone clearance after shock wave lithotripsy or ureteroscopy: the impact of lower pole radiographic anatomy. J Urol 159: 676–682
12. Elbahnasy AM, Clayman RV, Shalhav AL, Hoenig DM, Chandhoke P, Lingeman JE, Denstedt JD, Kahn R, Assimos DG, Nakada SY (1998) Lower-pole caliceal stone

clearance after shockwave lithotripsy, percutaneous nephrolithotomy, and flexible ureteroscopy: impact of radiographic spatial anatomy. J Endourol 12:113–119

13. Hubner W, Porpaczy P (1990) Treatment of caliceal calculi. Br J Urol 66:9–11

14. Lingeman JE, Newman D, Mertz JH, Mosbaugh PG, Steele RE, Kahnoski RJ, Coury TA, Woods JR (1986) Extracorporeal shock wave lithotripsy: the Methodist Hospital of Indiana experience. J Urol 135:1134–1137

15. Lingeman JE, Woods J, Toth PD, Evan AP, McAteer JA (1989) The role of lithotripsy and its side effects. J Urol 141:793–797

16. Vallancien G, Defourmestraux N, Leo JP, Cohen L, Puissan J, Veillon B, Brisset JM (1988) Outpatient extracorporeal lithotripsy of kidney stones: 1200 treatments. Eur Urol 15:1–4

17. Graff J, Diederichs W, Schulze H (1988) Long-term followup in 1003 extracorporeal shock wave lithotripsy patients. J Urol 140:479–483

18. Drach GW, Dretler SP, Fair W, Finlayson B, Gillenwater J, Griffith D, Lingeman JE, Newman D (1986) Report of the United States cooperative study of extracorporeal shock wave lithotripsy. J Urol 135:1127–1133

19. Chaussy C, Brendel W, Schmiedt E (1980) Extracorporeally induced destruction of kidney stones by shock waves. Lancet 2:1265–1268

20. Politis G, Griffin DP (1987) ESWS: stone-free efficacy based upon stone size and location. World J Urol 5:255

21. Roth RA, Beckmann CF (1988) Complications of extracorporeal shock-wave lithotripsy and percutaneous nephrolithotomy. Urol Clin North Am 15:155–166

22. Coptcoat MJ, Webb DR, Kellett MJ, Fletcher MS, McNicholas TA, Dickinson IK, Whitfield HN, Wickham JE (1986) The complications of extracorporeal shockwave lithotripsy: management and prevention. Br J Urol 58:578–580

23. Tolon M, Miroglu C, Erol H, Tolon J, Acar D, Bazmanoglu E, Erkan A, Amato S (1991) A report on extracorporeal shock wave lithotripsy results on 1569 renal units in an outpatient clinic. J Urol 145:695–698

24. Psihramis KE, Jewett MA, Bombardier C, Caron D, Ryan M (1992) Lithostar extracorporeal shock wave lithotripsy: the first 1000 patients. Toronto Lithotripsy Assoc J Urol 147:1006–1009

25. Motola JA, Smith AD (1990) Therapeutic options for the management of upper tract calculi. Urol Clin North Am 17:191–206

26. Graff J, Benkert S, Pastor J, Senge T (1989) Experience with a new multifunctional lithotripter, the Dornier MFL 5000: results of 415 treatments. J Endourol 3: 315–319

27. Lingeman JE, Coury TA, Newman DM, Kahnoski RJ, Mertz JH, Mosbaugh PG, Steele RE, Woods JR (1987) Comparison of results and morbidity of percutaneous nephrostolithotomy and extracorporeal shock wave lithotripsy. J Urol 138:485–490

28. Fedullo LM, Pollack HM, Banner MP, Amendola MA, Van Arsdalen KN (1988) The development of steinstrassen after ESWL: frequency, natural history, and radiologic management. Am J Roentgenol 151:1145–1147

29. Van Arsdalen KV (1987) Adjunctive procedures for ESWL. AUA Update Series 6:2

30. Chaussy CG, Fuchs GJ (1987) Extracorporeal shock wave lithotripsy of distal–ureteral calculi: is it worthwhile? J Endourol 1:1–8

31. Bregg K, Riehle RA Jr (1989) Morbidity associated with indwelling internal ureteral stents after shock wave lithotripsy. J Urol 141:510–512

32. Saltzman B (1988) Ureteral stents. Indications, variations, and complications (review). Urol Clin North Am 15:481–491

33. Shabsigh R, Gleeson MJ, Griffith DP (1988) The benefits of stenting on a more-or-less routine basis prior to extracorporeal shock-wave lithotripsy. Urol Clin North Am 15:493–497
34. Riehle RA Jr (1988) Selective use of ureteral stents before extracorporeal shock-wave lithotripsy. Urol Clin North Am 15:499–506
35. Segura JW (1987) Use and abuse of stents in the management of upper tract calculus disease. Probl Urol 7:649
36. Lee MH, Lee YH, Chen MT, Huang JK, Chang LS (1990) Management of painful caliceal stones by extracorporeal shock wave lithotripsy. Eur Urol 18:211–214
37. Netto NR, Claro JF, Lemos GC, Cortado PL (1991) Treatment options for ureteral calculi: endourology or extracorporeal shock wave lithotripsy. J Urol 146:5–7
38. McDougall EM, Denstedt JD, Brown RD, Clayman RV, Preminger GM, McClennan BL (1989) Comparison of extracorporeal shock wave lithotripsy and percutaneous nephrolithotomy for the treatment of renal calculi in lower pole calices. J Endourol 3:265–271
39. Dretler SP (1988) Stone fragility—a new therapeutic distinction. J Urol 139:1124–1127
40. Khan SR, Hackett RL, Finlayson B (1986) Morphology of urinary stone particles resulting from ESWL treatment. J Urol 136:1367–1372
41. Zhong P, Preminger GM (1994) Mechanisms of differing stone fragility in extracorporeal shockwave lithotripsy. J Endourol 8:263–268
42. Spirnak JP, Resnick MI (eds) (1990) Extracorporeal shock wave lithotripsy. In: Urolithiasis: a medical and surgical reference. Saunders, Philadelphia
43. Segura JW (1990) Current surgical approaches to nephrolithiasis. Endocrinol Metab Clin North Am 19:919–935
44. Lingeman JE, Siegel YI, Steele B, Nyhuis AW, Woods JR (1994) Management of lower pole nephrolithiasis: a critical analysis. J Urol 151:663–667
45. Lingeman JE, Lower Pole Study Group (1997) Prospective randomized trial of extracorporeal shock wave lithotripsy and percutaneous nephrostolithotomy for lower pole nephrolithiasis: initial long-term follow-up. J Endourol 11:S95
46. Meretyk S, Bigg S, Clayman RV, Kavoussi LR, McClennan BL (1992) Caveat emptor: caliceal stones and the missing calix. J Urol 147:1091–1095
47. Munver R, Delvecchio FC, Preminger GM (1999) Supracostal access for percutaneous renal surgery: is it safe? J Urol 161:377S
48. Karlin GS, Smith AD (1989) Approaches to the superior calix: renal displacement technique and review of options. J Urol 142:774–777
49. Bagley DH (1993) Intrarenal access with the flexible ureteropyeloscope: effects of active and passive tip deflection. J Endourol 7:221–224
50. Kuo RL, Aslan P, Zhong P, Preminger GM (1998) Impact of holmium laser settings and fiber diameter on stone fragmentation and endoscope deflection. J Endourol 12:523–527
51. Kourambas J, Delvecchio FC, Preminger GM (2000) Nitinol stone retrieval-assisted ureteroscopic management of lower pole renal calculi. Urology 56:935–939
52. Honey RJ (1998) Assessment of a new tipless nitinol stone basket and comparison with an existing flat-wire basket. J Endourol 12:529–531
53. Puppo P, Bottino P, Germinale F, Caviglia C, Ricciotti G, Giuliani L (1990) Flexible antegrade and retrograde nephroscopy: review of 50 cases. Eur Urol 17:193–199

54. Bagley DH (1990) Removal of upper urinary tract calculi with flexible ureteropyeloscopy. Urology 35:412–416
55. Abdel-Razzak OM, Bagley DH (1992) Clinical experience with flexible ureteropyeloscopy. J Urol 148:1788–1792
56. Fuchs AM, Fuchs GJ (1990) Retrograde intrarenal surgery for calculus disease: new minimally invasive treatment approach. J Endourol 4:337–345
57. Grasso M, Ficazzola M (1999) Retrograde ureteropyeloscopy for lower pole caliceal calculi [see comments]. J Urol 162:1904–1908
58. Kuo RL, Aslan P, Fitzgerald KB, Preminger GM (1998) Use of ureteroscopy and holmium: YAG laser in patients with bleeding diatheses. Urology 52: 609–613
59. Hofbauer J, Hobarth K, Marberger M (1992) Lithoclast: new and inexpensive mode of intracorporeal lithotripsy. J Endourol 6:429–432
60. Denstedt JD, Eberwein PM, Singh RR (1992) The Swiss lithoclast: a new device for intracorporeal lithotripsy. J Urol 148:1088–1090
61. Zhu S, Kourambas J, Munver R, Zhong P, Preminger GM (2000) Characterization of tip movement of the lithoclast flexible probe. J Urol 163(4S):318
62. Clayman RV, Kavoussi LR, Soper NJ, Dierks SM, Meretyk S, Darcy MD, Roemer FD, Pingleton ED, Thomson PG, Long SR (1991) Laparoscopic nephrectomy: initial case report. J Urol 146:278–282
63. Winfield HN, Donovan JF, Godet AS, Clayman RV (1993) Laparoscopic partial nephrectomy: initial case report for benign disease. J Endourol 7:521–526
64. Gaur DD, Agarwal DK, Purohit KC, Darshane AS (1994) Retroperitoneal laparoscopic pyelolithotomy. J Urol 151:927–929
65. Gluckman GR, Stoller ML, Irby P (1993) Laparoscopic pyelocaliceal diverticula ablation. J Endourol 7:315–317
66. Ruckle HC, Segura JW (1994) Laparoscopic treatment of a stone-filled, caliceal diverticulum: a definitive, minimally invasive therapeutic option. J Urol 151: 122–124
67. Redman JF (1983) Partial nephrectomy. Urol Clin North Am 10:677–684
68. Andersson L, Sylven M (1983) Small renal caliceal calculi as a cause of pain. J Urol 130:752–753
69. Brannen GE, Bush WH, Lewis GP (1986) Caliceal calculi. J Urol 135:1142–1145
70. Mee SL, Thuroff JW (1988) Small caliceal stones: is extracorporeal shock wave lithotripsy justified? J Urol 139:908–910
71. Netto NR Jr, Claro JF, Ferreira U, Lemos GC (1989) Small caliceal stones: what is the best method of treatment? J Urol 142:941–942
72. Netto NR, Claro JF, Lemos GC, Cortado PL (1991) Renal calculi in lower pole calices: what is the best method of treatment? J Urol 146:721–723
73. Netto NR, Claro JF, Cortado PL, Lemos GC (1991) Adjunct controlled inversion therapy following extracorporeal shock wave lithotripsy for lower pole caliceal stones. J Urol 146:953–954
74. Brownlee N, Foster M, Griffith DP, Carlton CE Jr (1990) Controlled inversion therapy: an adjunct to the elimination of gravity-dependent fragments following extracorporeal shock wave lithotripsy. J Urol 143:1096–1098
75. Nicely ER, Maggio MI, Kuhn EJ (1992) The use of a cystoscopically placed cobra catheter for directed irrigation of lower pole caliceal stones during extracorporeal shock wave lithotripsy. J Urol 148:1036–1039

76. Graham JB, Nelson JB (1994) Percutaneous caliceal irrigation during extracorporeal shock wave lithotripsy for lower pole renal calculi. J Urol 152:2227
77. Kourambas J, Delvecchio FC, Kuo RL, Preminger GM (1999) Ureteroscopic management of recurrent renal cystine calculi. J Endourol 13:A122
78. Timmons JW Jr, Malek RS, Hattery RR, Deweerd JH (1975) Caliceal diverticulum. J Urol 114:6–9
79. Middleton AW Jr, Pfister RC (1974) Stone-containing pyelocaliceal diverticulum: embryogenic, anatomic, radiologic and clinical characteristics. J Urol 111:2–6
80. Burns JR (1992) Calyceal diverticulum. AUA Updates Series XL(6):421
81. Psihramis KE, Dretler SP (1987) Extracorporeal shock wave lithotripsy of caliceal diverticula calculi. J Urol 138:707–711
82. Ritchie AW, Parr NJ, Moussa SA, Tolley DA (1990) Lithotripsy for calculi in caliceal diverticula? Br J Urol 66:6–8
83. Jones JA, Lingeman JE, Steidle CP (1991) The roles of extracorporeal shock wave lithotripsy and percutaneous nephrostolithotomy in the management of pyelocaliceal diverticula. J Urol 146:724–727
84. Streem SB, Yost A (1992) Treatment of caliceal diverticular calculi with extracorporeal shock wave lithotripsy: patient selection and extended followup. J Urol 148: 1043–1046
85. Hendrikx AJ, Bierkens AF, Bos R, Oosterhof GO, Debruyne FM (1992) Treatment of stones in caliceal diverticula: extracorporeal shock wave lithotripsy versus percutaneous nephrolitholapaxy. Br J Urol 70:478–482
86. Hulbert JC, Reddy PK, Hunter DW, Castaneda-Zuniga W, Amplatz K, Lange PH (1986) Percutaneous techniques for the management of caliceal diverticula containing calculi. J Urol 135:225–227
87. Bellman GC, Silverstein JI, Blickensderfer S, Smith AD (1993) Technique and follow-up of percutaneous management of caliceal diverticula. Urology 42:21–25
88. Fuchs GJ, David RD (1989) Flexible ureterorenoscopy, dilatation of narrow caliceal neck, and ESWL: a new, minimally invasive approach to stones in caliceal diverticula. J Endourol 3:255–263
89. Grasso M, Lang G, Loisides P, Bagley D, Taylor F (1995) Endoscopic management of the symptomatic caliceal diverticular calculus. J Urol 153:1878–1881
90. Soucie JM, Coates RJ, McClellan W, Austin H, Thun M (1996) Relation between geographic variability in kidney stones prevalence and risk factors for stones. Am J Epidemiol 143:487–495
91. Pak CY, Resnick MI, Preminger GM (1997) Ethnic and geographic diversity of stone disease. Urology 50:504–507
92. Soucie JM, Thun MJ, Coates RJ, McClellan W, Austin H (1994) Demographic and geographic variability of kidney stones in the United States. Kidney Int 46:893–899
93. Milliner DS, Murphy ME (1993) Urolithiasis in pediatric patients. Mayo Clin Proc 68:241–248
94. Chow GK, Streem SB (1998) Contemporary urological intervention for cystinuric patients: immediate and long-term impact and implications. J Urol 160: 341–345
95. Chow GK, Streem SB (1996) Medical treatment of cystinuria: results of contemporary clinical practice. J Urol 156:1576–1578
96. Gupta M, Bolton DM, Stoller ML (1995) Etiology and management of cystine lithiasis. Urology 45:344–355

97. Koide T, Yoshioka T, Yamaguchi S, Utsunomiya M, Sonoda T (1992) A strategy of cystine stone management. J Urol 147:112–114

98. Linari F, Marangella M, Fruttero B (1980) The natural history of cystinuria: A 15-year follow-up in 106 patients. In: Urolithiasis: clinical and basic research. Plenum Press, New York, pp 145–148

99. Kachel TA, Vijan SR, Dretler SP (1991) Endourological experience with cystine calculi and a treatment algorithm. J Urol 145:25–28

100. Katz G, Kovalski N, Landau EH (1993) Extracorporeal shock wave lithotripsy for treatment of ureterolithiasis in patients with cystinuria. Br J Urol 72:13–16

101. Katz G, Lencovsky Z, Pode D, Shapiro A, Caine M (1990) Place of extracorporeal shock-wave lithotripsy (ESWL) in management of cystine calculi. Urology 36:124–128

102. Hernandez-Graulau JM, Castaneda-Zuniga W, Hunter D, Hulbert JC (1989) Management of cystine nephrolithiasis by endourologic methods and shock-wave lithotripsy. Urology 34:139–143

103. Assimos DG (1996) Complications of stone removal. In: Smith AD, Badlani GH, Bagley DH, Clayman RV, Jordan GH, Kavoussi LR, Lingeman JE, Preminger GM, Segura JW (eds) Smith's Textbook of Endourology. Quality Medical Publishing, St. Louis, pp 298–308

104. Lechevallier E, Siles S, Ortega JC, Coulange C (1993) Comparison by SPECT of renal scars after extracorporeal shock wave lithotripsy and percutaneous nephrolithotomy. J Endourol 7:465–467

105. Dretler SP (1990) An evaluation of ureteral laser lithotripsy: 225 consecutive patients. J Urol 143:267–272

106. Wu TT, Hsu TH, Chen MT, Chang LS (1993) Efficacy of in vitro stone fragmentation by extracorporeal, electrohydraulic, and pulsed-dye laser lithotripsy. J Endourol 7:391–393

107. Grasso M, Conlin M, Bagley D (1998) Retrograde ureteropyeloscopic treatment of 2cm or greater upper urinary tract and minor Staghorn calculi. J Urol 160: 346–351

108. Moon YT, Kim SC (1993) Fate of clinically insignificant residual fragments after extracorporeal shock wave lithotripsy with EDAP LT-01 lithotripter. J Endourol 7:453–456

109. Van Horn AC, Hollander JB, Kass EJ (1995) First and second generation lithotripsy in children: results, comparison and followup. J Urol 153:1969–1971

110. Beck EM, Riehle RA Jr (1991) The fate of residual fragments after extracorporeal shock wave lithotripsy monotherapy of infection stones. J Urol 145: 6–10

111. Eisenberger F, Bub P, and Schmidt A (1992) The fate of residual fragments after extracorporeal shock wave lithotripsy. J Endourol 6:217–218

112. Newman DM, Scott JW, Lingeman JE (1988) Two-year follow-up of patients treated with extracorporeal shock wave lithotripsy. J Endourol 2:163–171

113. Streem SB, Yost A, Mascha E (1996) Clinical implications of clinically insignificant stone fragments after extracorporeal shock wave lithotripsy. J Urol 155: 1186–1190

114. Krings F, Tuerk C, Steinkogler I, Marberger M (1992) Extracorporeal shock wave lithotripsy retreatment ("stir-up") promotes discharge of persistent caliceal stone fragments after primary extracorporeal shock wave lithotripsy. J Urol 148: 1040–1042

115. Parr NJ, Ritchie AW, Smith G, Moussa SA, Tolley DA (1991) Does further extracorporeal lithotripsy promote clearance of small residual fragments? Br J Urol 68: 565–567
116. Cicerello E, Merlo F, Fandella A, Baggio B, Anselmo G (1994) Effect of alkaline citrate therapy on clearance of residual renal stone fragments after extracorporeal shock wave lithotripsy in sterile calcium and infection nephrolithiasis patients. J Urol 151:5–9
117. Fine JK, Pak CY, Preminger GM (1995) Effect of medical management and residual fragments on recurrent stone formation following shock wave lithotripsy. J Urol 153:27–33

Urolithiasis in Children—ESWL and Auxiliary Measures

PETER-MARTIN BRAUN, JEANETTE HOANG-BÖHM, and PETER ALKEN

Summary. In general, the criteria for the treatment of urolithiasis in children are the same as those for adults. Today, extracorporeal shockwave lithotripsy (ESWL) is the method of choice in the treatment of most pediatric urinary stones. Stone-free rates between 67% and 93% at short-term follow-up, and between 57% and 92% at long-term follow-up have proved the efficacy of ESWL treatment in children. Nevertheless, the demand for auxiliary measures still remains. In order to achieve the most beneficial success rates with few complications, it is advisable to perform this type of ESWL in centers that have the experience necessary for ESWL and endourological measures in children.

Key Words. ESWL in children, Stone-free rate, Auxiliary measures

Introduction

Since the introduction of extracorporeal shockwave lithotripsy (ESWL) by Chaussy in 1980, the therapeutic strategy for urolithiasis has completely changed. Nowadays, 96% of all urinary stones can be treated successfully by ESWL. In 1986, Newman et al. [1] published the first reports on ESWL in children. Since then, numerous further reports have been published on the effectivity and safety of ESWL in children [1–31]. In contrast to adults, only 1% to 3% of all urinary stones are detected in children. As a result, extensive experience in ESWL treatment in children is demanded at all stone centers. Therefore, the number of patients enrolled in each individual study varies between 1 and 73 [7, 24, 25, 30, 32–36]. One overall survey has been made on 446 children in over 250 stone centers [25]. Very few reports have been published that pro-

Department of Urology, Klinikum Mannheim gGmbH of the University of Heidelberg, D-68135 Mannheim, Germany

vide exact statistics on the frequency of auxiliary measures in children [7, 25, 30, 32–34, 36].

Interesting Aspects of ESWL in Children

Calyceal or renal stones with a stone diameter of up to 2 cm are an ideal indication for ESWL. More effective disintegration of even larger stones, together with swifter and uncomplicated discharge of larger concrements, can be achieved in children by ESWL. Consequently, ESWL can be indicated in children with a larger stone volume, and the placement of a ureteral stent before or after ESWL is generally unnecessary [9, 21, 29, 34].

In our series of 46 children, staghorn stones were detected in 20%, renal stones with a diameter of over 1.5 cm in 34%, and calyceal stones with a diameter of 0.3–2.0 cm in 29% [7, 32]. A further indication for ESWL in combination with endoscopic measures are proximal and distal ureteral stones that do not pass spontaneously [9, 10]. However, potential damage of the gonadal tissue in the ovaries caused by ESWL is still a controversial subject, and ESWL in female infants is considered a contraindication by several authors.

Lithotriptor Modifications

In principle, the same ESWL procedure is performed for both children and adults. Specific modifications depend on the age and size of the child and also on the type of lithotriptor in use. With the Dornier HM3 (Dornier Med Tech, Gemering, Germany), a polystyrene shield was used as lung protection in children smaller than 120 cm [14, 27–29, 34]. Nowadays, no additional equipment is needed in the treatment of infants and babies on 2nd- and 3rd-generation lithotriptors [2, 7, 20, 21, 23, 25, 32, 36–38] (Fig. 1). The waterbath of the HM3 has

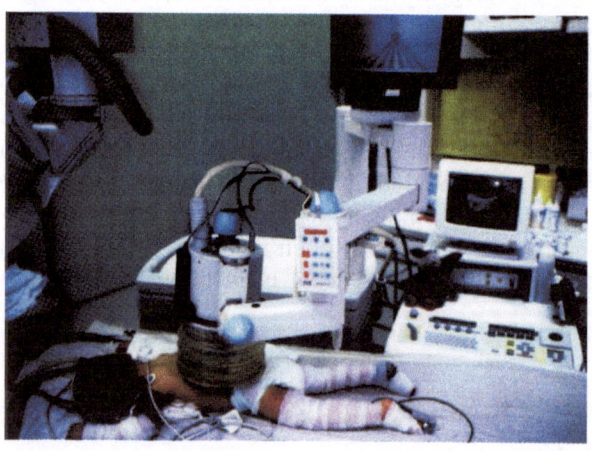

Fig. 1. A 12-month-old child being treated with the Modulith SLK (Storz Medical AG, Kreuzlingen, Germany)

been replaced by a multifunctional table that allows better positioning of children and uncomplicated treatment in supine and prone positions. The ultrasound location systems and digital fluoroscopy allow precise location of the stones at lower radiation exposure. The fluoroscopic screening times in children during treatment for renal stones averages 2.6 min, and that for ureteral stones averages 3.0 min [25].

The average radiation exposure for children is 106.6 (16–415) cGy/cm^2, which is considerably lower than the 250 cGy/cm^2 for adults [11]. A further attribute of the new lithotriptors allows the precise focusing of energy on the stone, thus minimizing potential tissue damage.

Anesthesia

Although, nowadays, no general anesthetic is normally administered to adults for ESWL treatment, this is not the case with children. A general anesthetic is demanded in 30% to 100% of children treated by ESWL. However, this demand, together with the method of anesthesia, varies strongly depending on the age of the child and type of lithotriptor in use. The reluctant cooperation of small infants when conscious makes a general anesthetic advisable in this group [2, 3, 11, 13, 14, 19, 24, 25, 39]. The age limit for analgosedation or no anesthetic at all in children treated by modern lithotriptors varies between 3 years (Piezolith) and 12 years (HM3) [21, 29, 36, 40]. In our department, children up to the age of 8 years treated by ESWL were routinely given a general anesthetic or preferably, if possible, analgosedation. Only poor compliance necessitated general anesthetics in older children. General anesthesia was administered to 30 out of 46 children (aged 3 months to 14 years). Sixteen children received analgosedation (aged 14–17 years). ESWL was performed with the Lithostar Plus (Siemens AG, Erlangen, Germany) and the Modulith SL20/SLX and SLK (Storz Medical AG, Kreuzlingen, Switzerland) (Fig. 1).

Disintegration and Stone-Free Rates

In the past, the chief aim of stone surgery was to achieve a complete stone-free condition. Although this does not quite apply to ESWL, long-term success depends on the stone-free rate. Complete stone disintegration is achieved in 57% to 97% of cases [1–31], but this is still only a prerequisite for a stone-free condition. In contrast to adults, more effective disintegration by ESWL and subsequent swifter and uncomplicated passage of larger concrements has frequently been observed in children [9, 21, 32, 34]. The reasons for this could be that, in general, the dwelling time of stones in children is only short, the shockwave effect is stronger in children, and they also quickly recuperate [34] from this method of treatment. After ESWL, 37% to 52% of the children were stone-free at discharge [7, 11, 29, 32], and the stone-free rate was between 57% and 97% three months after treatment [1–31].

TABLE 1. Stone-free rate and auxiliary measures in different studies

Study	Number of patients	Stone-free rate (%) after 3–6 months	Auxiliary measures (%)
Nijman et al. (34)	73	79	
Vandeursen et al. (36)	28	90.5	
Moreno et al. (33)	14	71.4	14.28
Zanetti et al. (30)	14	92.85	
Moazam (39)	83	82	
Myers et al. (25)	446	Kidney 67.9; Ureter 91.1	kidney 36.3; Ureter 17.7
Nazh et al. (35)	67	88.6	9
Own series	46	81	Adjuvant 19.6; Curative 8.7

Auxiliary Measures

The demand for pre- and posttherapeutic auxiliary measures is lower in infants than in older children or adults [11, 21–23, 27–29, 34, 38] (Table 1). Large concrements are often easily discharged by infants, thus making stent insertion unnecessary [36]. In principle, the auxiliary measures for urinary diversion in complicated hydronephrosis, e.g., ureteral stent and percutaneous nephrostomy (PCN), together with those for stone removal, e.g., uretrorenoscopy (URS) and percutaneous nephrolithoapaxy (PCNL), are usually defined as overall auxiliary measures [14, 41]. However, a distinction must be made, for both adults and children, between these two groups of auxiliary measures. *Curative* auxiliary measures aim at a stone-free condition. These comprise lithotripsy and stone extraction by ureterorenoscopy and PCNL, respectively. Those measures with an *adjuvant* effect attempt to suppress complications to a minimum, and include the insertion of ureteral stents or percutaneous nephrostomies. Curative auxiliary measures are invasive and must be carried out under general anesthetic in both younger and older children. Adjuvant measures are less invasive and can frequently be performed under analgosedation. Of our young patients, 19.6% were treated by adjuvant auxiliary procedures and 8.7% by curative auxiliary measures [7, 32]. Information on auxiliary measures is rarely given in the literature— the frequency is reported to be 14% to 37% [25, 33–35, 39]. It must never be forgotten that retrograde auxiliary measures over ureterorenoscopy in boys always entails the risk of damage to the urethra, with subsequent urethral strictures. Hence, whenever possible, this procedure should be avoided in the treatment of boys. Instead, it is advisable either to repeat ESWL, or to use antegrade procedures over PCNL. In our group of patients, ureterorenoscopy was needed only once for a distal ureteral stone in a small boy.

Complications

Petechiea bleeding on the skin or slight hematuria often arise, although severe complications after ESWL are less frequent in children than in adults. The complication rate lies between 6% and 26% [2, 3, 11, 25, 29, 38]. Urinary tract infection accompanied by a high temperature up to sepsis is the most common complication that originates from previously existing, persistent urinary tract infection. The complication rate in our series of patients was 8%, and these were all episodes of high temperature from previously existing, persistent urinary tract infection caused by obstruction of the upper urinary tract. These complications were all conservatively managed by percutaneous procedures or retrograde ureteral stents plus additional antibiotic therapy [7, 32]. Very severe complications that can arise in connection with the infantile anatomical structure, e.g., pulmonary contusion, hemoptysis, or perirenal hematoma, have only been described in reports on four series of patients [2, 13, 14, 27].

Long-Term Results

Stone-Free Rate and Stone Recurrence Rate

Only five reports [8, 11, 18, 19, 29] have been published on stone-free rates in children. These showed rates between 57% and 92% in a long-term follow-up between 18 and 46 months after ESWL treatment. A general recurrence rate of between 2% and 44% has been given for children after ESWL [18, 29, 34, 42], and the residual fragment rate is between 23% and 33% [29, 34]. In contrast, the recurrence rate in adults is between 8% and 10%, and residual stone growth averages 22% [41]. Complex etiology, a high rate of metabolism disturbances, anatomical changes, and urinary tract infection are given as the reasons for the higher rate of residual stone growth in children [8, 42]. Of our small patients, 72% were stone-free after an average of 46 months, and 5/42 (13.7%) of these developed recurring stones. Residual stone growth progressed in all nine children who were *not* stone-free after 3 months. In all cases, urinary tract infection, metabolic disturbance, or an anatomical change was detected in those children suffering from stone recurrence or residual stone growth [7, 32].

Conclusion

Infant stone patients must be followed over a prolonged period in order to assess the safety and effectiveness of the treatment strategy. Sonographic and/or X-ray monitoring of the affected kidney should be performed at least 2 weeks and 3 months after ESWL. Any remaining stubborn residual concrements are then disintegrated in repeated ESWL treatment.

A metaphylaxis for metabolical disturbances and a long-term antibiosis for chronic infection is recommended in an attempt to avoid residual stones. Any existing infrarenal obstruction must first be cleared.

In order to achieve the greatest success rates with few complications, it is advisable to perform this type of ESWL in centers that have the experience necessary for ESWL and endourological measures in children.

References

1. Newman DM, Coury T, Lingeman JE, Mertz JHO, Mosbaugh PG, Steele RE, Knapp PM (1986) Extracorporeal shock wave lithotripsy experience in children. J Urol 136:238–240
2. Abara E, Merguerian PA, McLorie GA, Psihramis KE, Jewett MA, Churchill BM (1990) Lithostar extracorporeal shock wave lithotripsy in children. J Urol 144:489–493
3. Adams MC, Newman DM, Lingeman JE (1989) Pediatric ESWL: long-term results and effects on renal growth. J Endourol 3:245–254
4. Androulakakis PA (1992) Treatment of renal stones in children. Eur Urol Update Ser 1:50–54
5. Boddy SA, Kellett MJ, Fletcher MS, Ransley AMI, Paris AM, Whitfield HN, Wickham JF (1987) Extracorporeal shock wave lithotripsy and percutaneous nephrolithotomy in children. J Pediatr Surg 22:223–227
6. Bohle A, Knipper A, Thomas S (1989) Extracorporeal shock wave lithotripsy in pediatric patients. Scand J Urol Nephrol 23:137–140
7. Braun PM, Hoang-Böhm J, Esen T, Krautschick A, Alken P (1998) Therapy of urolithiasis in childhood—ESWL and auxiliary measures. Eur Urol 33(Suppl 1): 105
8. Esen T, Bürger R, Witzsch U, Beetz R, Hohenfellner R (1992) Role of metabolic evaluation and specific prophylaxis in the long-term outcome of extracorporeal shock wave lithotripsy in children. J Endourol 6:305–308
9. Frick J, Köhle R, Kunit G (1988) Experience with extracorporeal shock wave lithotripsy in children. Eur Urol 14:181–183
10. Frick J, Sarica K, Kohle R, Kunit G (1991) Long-term follow-up after extracorporeal shockwave lithotripsy in children. Eur Urol 19:225–229
11. Gschwend JE, Paiss T, Gottfried HW, Hautmann RE (1995) Extrakorporale Stosswellenlithotripsie bei Kindern. Komplikationen und Langzeitergebnisse. Urologe A 34:324–328
12. Harmon EP, Neal DE, Thomas R (1994) Pediatric urolithiasis: review of research and current management. Pediatr Nephrol 8:508–512
13. Kramolowsky EV, Willoughby BL, Loening SA (1987) Extracorporeal shock wave lithotripsy in children. J Urol 137:939–941
14. Kroovand RL, Harrison LH, McCullough DL (1987) Extracorporeal shock wave lithotripsy in children. J Urol 138:1106–1108
15. Kroovand RL (1992) Stones in pregnancy and in children. J Urol 148:1076–1178
16. Lee KW, Rodo-Salas J, Moralales-Fochs L (1995) Course of the urinary lithiasis treatment in the surgery department of a children's hospital. Cir Pediatr 8:47–50
17. Lim DJ, Walker RD, Ellsworth PI, Newman RC, Cohen MS, Barraza MA, Stevens PS (1996) Treatment of pediatric urolithiasis between 1984 and 1994. J Urol 156: 702–705
18. Lock MT, Speelmann A, Nijman JM, Ackaert KS, Dik P, Scholtmeijer RJ (1989) Experiences with extracorporeal shockwave lithotripsy in 61 children. Ned Tijdschr Geneeskd 133:669–672
19. Losty P, Surana R, O'Donnell B (1993) Limitations of extracorporeal shock wave lithotripsy for urinary tract calculi in young children. J Pediatr Surg 28:1037–1039
20. Lottmann H, Armchanbaud F, Helal B, Mercier-Pageyral B, Melin Y (1995) Extracorporeal shockwave lithotripsy in children. Study of the effectiveness and renal consequences in a series of eighteen children. Ann Urol Paris 29:136–142

21. Marberger M, Türk C, Steinkogler I (1989) Piezoelectric extracorporeal shock wave lithotripsy in children. J Urol 142:349–352
22. Mininberg D (1989) Extracorporeal shock wave lithotripsy in children: an overview. J Endourol 3:385–389
23. Miroglu C, Tokuc R, Erol H, Tolon J, Erkan A, Bazmanoglu E, Tolon M (1992) Extracorporeal shock wave lithotripsy in children: report on 79 renal units. J Endourol 6:209–211
24. Mishriki SF, Wills M, Mukherjee A, Frank JD, Feneley RCL (1992) Extracorporeal shock wave lithotripsy for renal calculi in children. Br J Urol 69:303–305
25. Myers DA, Mobley TB, Jenkins JM, Grine WB, Jordan WR (1995) Pediatric low-energy lithotripsy with the lithostar. J Urol 153:453–457
26. Sarica K, Kupei S, Sarica N, Gogus O, Kilic S, Saribas S (1995) Long-term follow-up of renal morphology and function in children after lithotripsy. Urol Int 54:95–98
27. Sigman M, Laudone VP, Jenkins AD, Howards SS, Riehle R, Keating MA, Walker RD (1987) Initial experience with extracorporeal shock wave lithotripsy in children. J Urol 138:839–841
28. Schultz-Lampel D, Lazica M, Lampel A, Thüroff JW (1991) ESWL treatment of urinary stones in children. J Endourol 5:S137
29. Schultz-Lampel D, Lazica M, Lampel A, Bohnen K, Thüroff JW (1994) Langzeitverlauf nach ESWL bei Kindern: Steinfreiheit, Rezidivsteinrate, Blutdruck und Nierenfunktion. Aktuel Urol 25:101–110
30. Zanetti GR, Montanari E, Guarneri A, et al. (1993) Extracorporeal shock wave lithotripsy with MPL 9000 for the treatment of urinary stones in pediatric patients. Arch Ital Urol Androl 65:671–673
31. Zöller G, Wassmann K, Ludewig M, Ringert R-H (1990) Extrakorporale Stosswellenlithotripsie eines Nierenbeckenausgusssteines bei einem 15 Monate alten Säugling. Aktuel Urol 21:210–213
32. Braun PM, Weber A, Michel MS, Spahn M, Köhrmann KU, Krautschick A, Alken P (1998) Are auxiliary measures necessary in therapy of urolithiasis in children? J Endourol 12(Suppl 1):P1–8
33. Moreno Aranda J, Cedillo Lopez U, Lopez Pelerano Jl, Hernandez Toriz N, Blanco Bernal SG (1992) Extracorporal lithotripsy in children. Gac Med Mex 128:263–266
34. Nijman JM, Ackaert K, Scholtmeijer RJ, Lock TWTM, Schröder FH (1989) Long-term results of extracorporeal shock wave lithotripsy in children. J Urol 142:609–611
35. Nazh O, Cal C, Özyurt C, Günaydin G, Cüreklibatir I, Avcieri V, Erhan O (1998) Results of extracorporeal shock wave lithotripsy in the pediatric age group. Eur Urol 33:333–336
36. Vandeursen H, Devos P, Baert L (1991) Electromagnetic shock wave lithotripsy in children. J Urol 145:1229–1231
37. Lin CM (1992) Extracorporeal shock wave lithotripsy in children: experience with the multifunctional lithotripter MFL 5000. Acta Pediatr Sin 33:357–362
38. Van Horn AC, Hollander JB, Kass EJ (1995) First and second generation lithotripsy in children: results, comparison and follow-up. J Urol 153:1969–1971
39. Moazam F, Nazir Z, Jafarey AM (1994) Pediatric urolithiasis: to cut or not to cut. J Pediatr Surg 29:761–764
40. Carvajal-Busslinger MI, Gygi C, Ackermann D, Kaiser G, Bianchetti M (1994) Urolithiasis in childhood. When do what? Eur J Pediatr Surg 4:199–200
41. Rassweiler JJ, Köhrmann KU, Seemann O, Tschada R, Alken P (1996) Kidney stones: medical and surgical management. In: Coe FC, Favus MJ, Park YC, Parks CH,

Preminger GM (eds) Clinical comparison of ESWL. Lippincott Raven, Philadelphia, pp 571–603

42. Diamond DA, Menon M, Lee PH, Rickwood AMK, Johnston JH (1989) Etiological factors in pediatric stone recurrence. J Urol 142:606–608
43. Charbit L, Terdjman S, Gendreau MC, Guerin D, Quental P, Cukier J (1989) La litotricia extracorporea por ondas de choque en el nino. Arch Esp Urol 42(Suppl 1):71–73
44. Pearle MS, Clayman RV (1996) Outcome and selection of surgical therapies of stones in the kidney and ureter. In: Coe FC, Favus MJ, Park YC, Parks CH, Preminger GM (eds) Clinical comparison of ESWL. Lippincott Raven, Philadelphia, pp 709–755
45. Thomas R, Frentz J, Harmon E, Frentz G (1992) Effect of extracorporeal shock wave lithotripsy on renal function and body height in pediatric patients. J Urol 148:1064–1066
46. Thornhill JA, Moran K, Mooney EE, Sheehan S, Smith JM, Fitzpatrick JM (1990) Extracorporeal shock wave lithotripsy monotherapy for pediatric urinary calculi. Br J Urol 65:638–640
47. Tolon M, Miroglu C, Erol H, et al. (1991) A report on extracorporeal shock wave lithotripsy results on 1569 renal units in an outpatient clinic. J Urol 145:695–698
48. Van Arsdalen KN, Kurzweil S, Smith J, Levin RM (1991) Effect of lithotripsy on immature rabbit bone and kidney development. J Urol 146:213–216
49. Zhou ZY, Zheng SG (1991) Piezoelectric lithotripter in the treatment of pediatric calculi. Chin Med J Engl 104:728–731

Treatment of Complicated Urolithiasis

Seiichi Orikasa, Naomasa Ioritani, Yutaka Chiba, Senji Hoshi,
and Atsushi Fukuzaki

Summary. Patients who now require an open operation have complex calculous diseases, including structural anomalies of the urinary tract and impacted stones, submucosal calculus, and stone granulation associated with refractory ureteral strictures. Current approaches to these problems, and the reasons why impacted stones are not fragmented by extracorporeal shock wave lithotripsy (ESWL) are reviewed.

Submucosal calculi or stone granulation should be considered when standard ESWL fails, or when postureteroscopic strictures are so refractory that they require operative repair. Every effort should be made to prevent crystals from becoming embedded in the ureteral wall during ureteroscopic manipulation.

Key Words. Complex calculus, Impacted calculus, Submucosal calculus, Stone granulation, Underwater shock wave

Introduction

During the last 20 years, significant advances in the treatment of urinary tract calculi have diminished the need for open operative management. Most renal and ureteral calculi are now treated with extracorporeal shock wave lithotripsy (ESWL, Dornier Medical Systems, Inc., Marietta, GA, USA) and endourological procedures. The location, size, and chemical composition of the stone, the patient's general health, and also all the advantages and disadvantages of ESWL, percutaneous nephrolithotomy (PNL), or transurethral ureterolithotomy (TUL), will dictate which treatment modality should be used. Paik et al. [1] reported that the current rate of open stone surgery was only 5.4% of 780 cases, and that the indications for open surgical stone removal were a complex stone burden (55%), ESWL and endourology failure (29%), anatomical renal and ureteral

Department of Urology, Tohoku University School of Medicine, 1-1 Seiryo-machi, Aoba-ku, Sendai 980-8574, Japan

abnormalities (24%), morbid obesity, and comorbid medical disease (17%). Although improving skills with ESWL and endourology have diminished the role of open surgery more than ever, open operative management of urinary calculi continues to represent a reasonable alternative in certain circumstances.

Here, current approaches to the complex calculous disease associated with a variety of anatomical and physiological problems are reviewed.

Anatomical Abnormalities of Kidney and Ureter

The majority of cases of horseshoe kidney and pelvic kidney, which are representative diseases of anomalous position and malrotation of the kidney, are managed successfully with ESWL or endourology, and open surgery is used infrequently. As an unusual example of an anomalous position of a kidney, a patient with a pelvic stone in a transplanted kidney was referred to our clinic. The stone was easily extracted with percutaneous manipulation because of the shallow position of the transplanted kidney in the pelvis (Fig. 1). The position of the kidney often deviates in patients with deformation of the spine due to spinal caries, spinal cord injury, or spinal curvature, etc. However, after the kidney is accurately located using computed tomography and ultrasonic examination, the majority of patients can be managed successfully with ESWL and/or PNL.

Other indications for an open operation include congenitally obstructed megaureter and ureteropelvic junction obstruction, with an inability to excrete

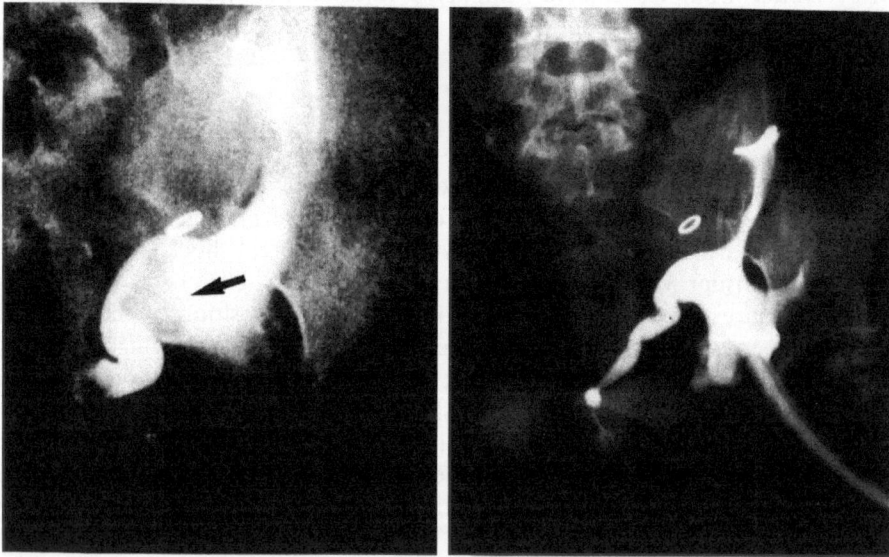

FIG. 1. Renal pelvic stone (*arrow*) in a transplanted kidney in a 29-year-old male was easily extracted by percutaneous nephrolithotomy

the fragments and to advance the endoscope. In some cases, however, it is possible to dilate and incise the stricture simultaneously using a dilator or laser, and subsequently to fragment the stone.

Impacted Stones

When ureteral calculi are impacted for more than 2 months in the same site, they frequently do not permit successful application of TUL or PNL because the stone cannot be directly observed endoscopically, even if the endoscope is advanced into the neighborhood of the stone. They also show minimal or no response after multiple ESWL treatments. Calculi can be impacted by the surrounding characteristic edema, epithelial hyperplasia, or an inflammatory polyp, which all cause narrowing of the ureteral lumen above and below the calculus. A catheter or guide wire cannot be passed beyond the stone at the initial attempt either because the calculus adheres tightly to the ureter wall and there is no space between the wall and the calculus. Such calculi are called impacted stones [2]. Histological studies have revealed mucosal edema, urothelial hypertrophy, chronic inflammation, and interstitial fibrosis at the site of impaction. The management of impacted stones remains a challenge for the urologist.

Once the stone has been visualized, fragmentation can be initiated. Therefore, the initial objective should be to disimpact the stone so that standard techniques may be applied. Disimpaction maneuvers include laser excision of the polyp, high-pressure saline irrigation via a ureteral catheter, or placing an occlusion balloon catheter below the stone to allow for hydrodilation of the ureter, with a subsequent repeat attempt to pass through a guide wire or a rigid ureteroscope. It should then be possible to perform fragmentation in situ with a pulsed-dye laser or ultrasound lithotripter, or to push the stone up into the kidney with a catheter or ureteroscope. Once the stone is dislodged or fragmented, the ureteroscope is advanced through the area of impaction to examine the proximal ureter. Proximal ureter stones or kidney stones are subsequently treated by ESWL. During ureteroscopy, an inability to pass a guide wire reduces the safety margin and increases the possibility of bleeding, perforation, or creation of a false passage. The edematous ureter is prone to hemorrhage and injury, or perforation of the ureteral wall with even a gentle technique, resulting in a high incidence of stricture formation. Therefore, staged ureteroscopy, with placement of a stent before ureteroscopic extraction, should be considered as another potential option for impacted stones. This would not only facilitate access to the stone, but may substantially decrease edema surrounding the stone, and thereby reduce the chance of ureteral injury during ureteroscopic manipulation. If it is not clear whether the pathological changes within the ureter around impacted stone are cancerous or inflammatory changes, this should be checked by biopsy specimens.

However, there are calculi which cannot be fragmented by ESWL. Calculi which are composed of cystine or calcium oxalate monohydrate are less likely to

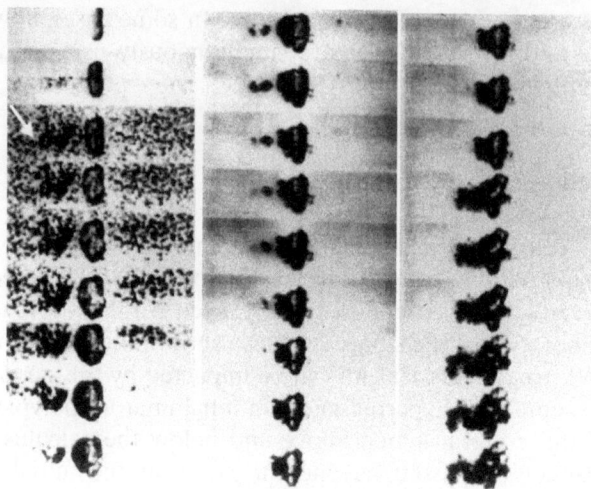

Fig. 2. High-speed cinematography, 6000 frames per second, of a process whereby a calcium oxalate stone suspended in gelatin was disintegrated by an underwater shock wave. The shock wave came from the left-hand side. The calculus is expanding and contracting repeatedly, and numerous cavitation bubbles (*arrow*) are also inflating and deflating repeatedly. The stone is then fragmented and blown out by the inflating cavitation inside it

respond to ESWL. Stones that appear dense on radiography are likely to be of the calcium oxalate monohydrate variety. In addition to the stone composition, there are other reasons why impacted stones are not fragmented by ESWL.

When the process of calculus disintegration by underwater shock waves was observed by high-speed photography, the calculi were seen to be expanding and contracting repeatedly, and also numerous cavitation bubbles around the focus were inflating and deflating repeatedly. The stone then seemed to be smashed into fragments and blown out by the inflating cavitation inside the stone [3] (Fig. 2). In this experiment, the stone was suspended in gelatin, whose acoustic impedance is almost equivalent to that of water. That is to say, in order to disintegrated the calculus by shock waves, expansion chambers are necessary. However, the impacted stone is completely surrounded by ureteral tissue, and there is no expansion chamber within the circumference of the calculus.

The decreased efficacy of ESWL for an unstented ureteral stone is well documented, and is presumably because of the lack of an adequate expansion chamber and a fluid–tissue interface. Fragmentation may be improved if a catheter is placed level with the stone, and saline is injected during ESWL to create a fluid–tissue interface, which thereby increases the effectiveness of the shock wave. The greater the difference in acoustic impedance between the calculus and the water, the easier it is for the calculus to be fragmented by the underwater shock wave. According to our data, the ratio of acoustic impedance of urinary calculi and human tissues to that of the water ranges from 2.4 to 3.7 and from 0.9 to 1.1, respectively [3]. In an impacted stone, water does not intervene between the ureter wall and the calculus, so that the difference in impedance between the calculus and the ureteral wall is less than that between the calculus and water, resulting in decrease in the fragmentation power of the shock waves. The power of the shock wave which reaches the calculus also decreases in an impacted stone because the ureter wall which is in contact with the calculus absorbs some of the power of the shock wave. Even though fractures develop within the stone, the stone–fluid interface does not increase and the central portion of the stone is not fragmented. Fragments confined by the ureter do not separate, and peripheral fragments continue to absorb the energy of the shock waves [4].

In addition to the fact that the calculus seems mainly to be disintegrated by the compressive and tensile forces of the shock wave, it is likely that the generation of a cavitation and microjet phenomenon, hammering water (rapid fluid streaming), and shearing forces generated by the underwater shock waves all play an important role during the fragmentation [3, 5, 6]. However, these effects are suppressed in an impacted stone, since water does not intervene between the calculus and the ureteral wall. These explanations have been deduced from our underwater fragmentation experiments using an agar plate (agar phantom) on the assumption of an impacted stone [7].

Despite the fact that the ratio of the acoustic impedance of the agar to that of water is 0.97, which is believed to be almost equivalent to that of soft tissue, a model stone (activated alumina, 6 mm in diameter) impacted inside a 1-cm-thick agar plate needed about three times as many shots of the underwater shock wave as stones in water before disintegration (Fig. 3A). When the 1-cm-thick agar plate was placed in the path of the shock waves and over 1 cm away from the stone, approximately 100% of the pressure of the shock waves was transmitted to the calculus, followed by its complete disintegration (Fig. 3B). However, the peak pressure behind the agar plate depended on the distance between the pressure transducer and the agar plate, and decreased markedly from a distance of 3 mm until it finally decreased to 87% at zero distance (Fig. 4). Therefore, when the agar was placed in contact with the calculus, the calculus hardly disintegrated at all (Fig. 3C). Figure 3A–C is believed to mimic the condition of an impacted stone, and the results suggest that an impacted stone decreases the effectiveness of the shock waves.

Submucosal Calculi and Stone Granulation

There are certain ureteral calculi that show minimal or no response after multiple ESWL treatments, and which are not visible during ureteroscopy, thus preventing endoscopic manipulation. These are submucosal calculi, of which microliths or fragments have migrated beneath the urothelium, and some have become the cause of a ureteral stricture due to stone granulation [8]. The reasons

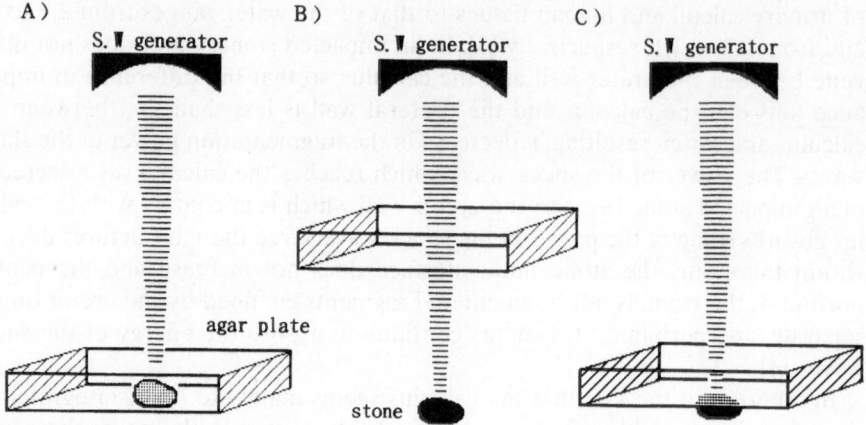

FIG. 3. Schematic diagram of experiments imitating an impacted stone. The acoustic impedance of the agar is almost equivalent to that of soft tissue. **A** An impacted stone inside the agar plate needed about three times as many underwater shock waves as a stone in water before it disintegrated. **B** If the agar plate was placed over 1 cm away from the stone, 100% of the pressure of the shock waves was transmitted through the agar to the stone. **C** When the agar plate was placed in contact with the stone, the pressure of the shock waves decreased and the stone hardly disintegrated at all

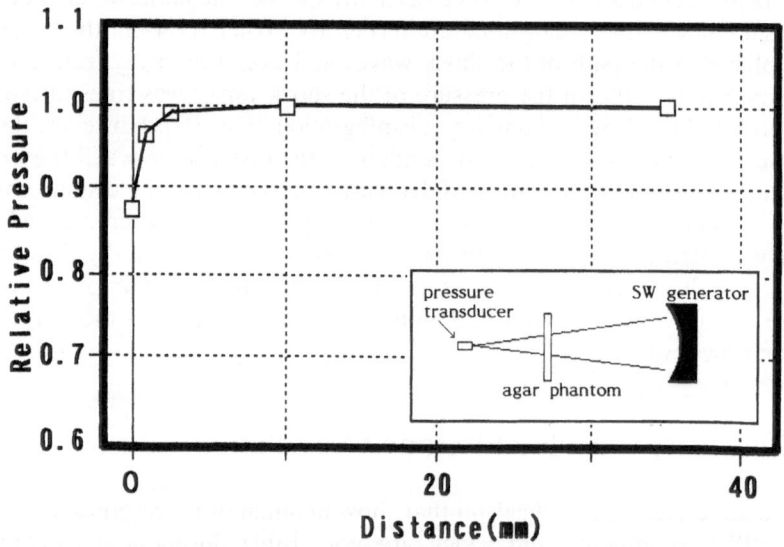

FIG. 4. The relative pressure behind the agar plate. Relative pressure depends on the distance between the pressure transducer and the agar plate, and decreases markedly from a distance of 3mm until it is only 87% at zero distance

why submucosal calculi are not fragmented by ESWL are the same as those for an impacted stone.

It is likely that the long-term presence of a calculus is necessary for submucosal migration to occur. Perhaps because of immobility and the persistent irritation caused by the calculus, a chronic inflammatory reaction could account for submucosal migration and epithelization over the stone. It may also be possible that stone manipulation and instrumentation to chronically inflamed ureteral mucosa may be all that is necessary to promote submucosal migration of the calculus. Stone fragments may be pushed into the disrupted area during fragmentation. Some fragments will be embedded in the perforated wall, and some will remain just outside the ureteral wall. Excessive use of ESWL energy may also result in ureteral injury.

When calculi under a thin mucosa can be confirmed by direct vision, it may be possible to extract the stone by ureteroscopy with mucosal incision. However, most fragments are not visible during ureteroscopy. Radiographically, one cannot distinguish whether the stone is intraluminal or buried in the submucosa (Fig. 5). Clinical signs and symptoms, including an obstruction above the stone on an excretory urogram coinciding with calcification on a plain film, frank pain, and gross or microscopic hematuria may not be different from the clinical features of normal ureteral calculi. Submucosal migration of chronic ureteral calculi should be considered when standard ESWL fails and no intraluminal stone can be located endoscopically.

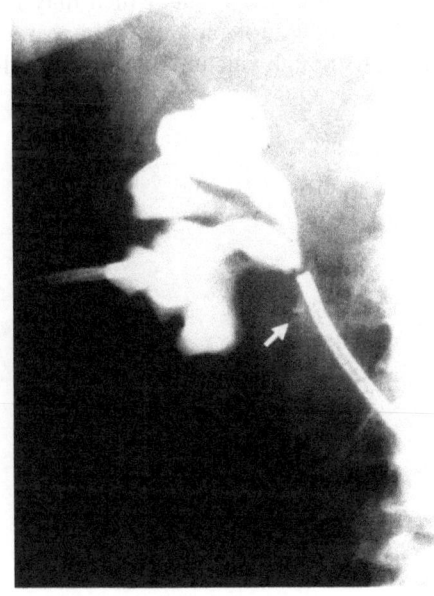

FIG. 5. Submucosal ureteral calculus. Antegrade pyelography with a ureteroscope in the ureter reveals stricture and extraluminal calcification (*arrow*). A 63-year-old man underwent percutaneous nephrolithotomy (PNL) using an electrohydraulic lithotripter for a ureteropelvic junction stone. This resulted in stricture 18 months later, coinciding with a calcification, as seen on plain film. Intra- or extraluminal stones cannot be distinguished on plain film

Although the mechanism of ureteral stricture formation has not yet been completely elucidated, and it is likely multifactorial, it has been generally assumed
that strictures associated with ureterocopy and stone fragmentation occur as a
direct result of localized mechanical ureteral trauma such as mucosal disruption,
false passage, perforation, and periureteral extravasation of urine. Thermal
injury due to ultrasound or a laser lithotripter, and relative ischemia from the
use of a large-diameter ureteroscope have also been implicated as contributory
factors in stricture formation. The refinement of existing technologies has led
to an overall decrease in the frequency of ureteral strictures associated with
ureteroscopy, and the rate of stricture formation at present is lower than 1%.
Although most of these strictures are successfully treated with ureteral dilation
or incision, some do not respond to endoscopic conservative management and
require operative repair.

If mucosal trauma was the sole cause of strictures requiring operative repair,
there would certainly have been many more strictures, and perforation alone is
unlikely to produce an irreversible fibrotic reaction. Dretler and Young [9] proposed that a new entity termed stone granulation should be suspected when postureteroscopic lithotripsy strictures are so refractory that they require operative
repair. During ureteroscopic stone fragmentation, calcium oxalate crystals are
embedded in the ureteral wall and result in persistent progressive foreign body
giant-cell reaction with fibrosis, which causes the occasional dense stricture.
Histologically, calcium oxalate crystals associated with macrophages, foreign
body giant cells, and a dense fibrotic reaction (stone granuloma) are seen in
fibrotic specimens (Fig. 6). Unlike calcium phosphate crystals that stain dark blue
with hematoxylin and eosin, calcium oxalate crystals stain light green and are
refractile, so they are not easily visible. The fixation process may even cause them
to fall out of the tissue, which may be the reason that ingested calcium oxalate
crystals have not previously been recognized in association with ureteral stricture. Although calcium oxalate monohydrate and dihydrate were found in stone

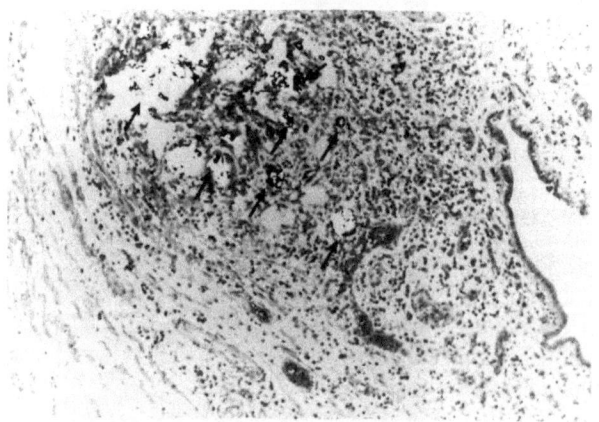

FIG. 6. Foreign body
granuloma containing
many crystallines fragments
(*arrows*), foreign body
giant cells, and
proliferation of
collagenized fibrous tissue.
H&E, reduced from ×300

granulation, it is not clear whether other crystal forms could induce a similar response. Motola et al. [10] described a similar pathological condition in three patients in whom endopyelotomy failed, and who then underwent open repair. Microscopic examination of surgical specimens revealed a foreign body granuloma that contained an intraluminal birefringent crystalline substance and the proliferation of dense collagenized fibrous materials. Roberts et al. [11] also reported that in two of five patients with ureteral stricture which had developed after intervention for an impacted stone, including four with and one without previous perforation, stone fragments were identified within the scar tissue at definitive endoscopic stone removal, and the pathology available in one case revealed chronic granulomatous giant-cell inflammation surrounding deposited calcium crystals in the ureter. No correlation between stricture formation and stone composition was found. Every effort should be made to prevent crystals from becoming embedded in the ureteral wall.

Infant and Morbid Obesity

The use of the ESWL equipment and endourology instruments is limited in infants and the morbidly obese. Open operations are preferabe for infants and children because there are frequent associated structural anomalies of the urinary tract such as congenital ureteropelvic junction obstruction or obstructed megaureter, and for economic efficiency. In a study by Lim et al. [12] 42% of patients had anatomical abnormalities and 25% underwent open surgery.

Although there are comparatively few such cases in Japan, open surgery is also done in cases of morbid obesity. Pregnant women and women of childbearing age are absolutely contraindicated for ESWL to avoid potential shock-wave-mediated ovarian or fetus injury.

Conclusion

A small group of patients develop complex calculous disease, including structural anomalies of the urinary tract and impacted stones, submucosal calculus, and stone granulation associated with refractory ureteral strictures. While successful therapy may often be achieved with minimum morbidity by a number of endourological methods as well as ESWL, these new therapeutic modalities may sometimes be much less effective and potentially associated with increased morbidity, so that open stone surgery continues to represent a reasonable alternative for such patients.

Since postureteroscopic strictures associated with stone granuloma are so refractory that they require operative repair, every effort should be made to prevent crystals from becoming embedded in the ureteral wall during ureteroscopic manipulation.

References

1. Paik MI, Wainstein MA, Spirnak JP, Hampel N, Resnick MI (1998) Current indications for open stone surgery in the treatment of renal and ureteral calculi. J Urol 159:374–379
2. Morgentaler A, Bridge SS, Dretler SP (1990) Management of the impacted ureteral calculus. J Urol 143:263–266
3. Kambe K, Kuwahara M, Orikasa S, Takayama K (1988) Mechanism of fragmentation of urinary stones by underwater shock wave. Urol Int 43:275
4. Parr NJ, Pye SD, Ritchie AWS, Tolley DA (1992) Mechanisms responsible for diminished fragmentation of ureteral calculi: an experimental and clinical study. J Urol 148:1079–1083
5. Kuwahara M, Kambe K, Ioritani N, Saito T, Shirai S, Orikasa S, Obara T, Takayama K, Aida S (1990) Mechanism of biological tissue injury induced by focused underwater shock waves: study on the cavitation and flow in the focused region. Proceedings of a Symposium on Shock Waves, Institute of Fluid Science, Tohoku University, Sendai, pp 7–12
6. Williams JC, Jr, Woodward JF, Stonehill MA, et al. (1999) Cell damage by lithotripter shock waves at high pressure to preclude cavitation. Ultrasound Med Biol 25:1445–1449
7. Aida S, Fujimoto K, Kuwahara M, Takayama K (1992) Experimental studies on the destructibility of impacted stones. Proceedings of the 18th International Symposium on Shock Waves, k11–12, Institute of Fluid Science, Tohoku University, Sendai (Proceedings of a Symposium on Shock Waves, Tokyo, 1990, pp 91–94)
8. Young MJ, Rubenstein MA, Norms DM, Lee RD, Moran GC (1990) Submucosal ureteral calculi: a new entity? J Urol 143:800–801
9. Dretler SP, Young RH (1993) Stone granuloma: a cause of ureteral stricture. J Urol 150:1800–1802
10. Motola JA, Badlani GH, Smith AD (1993) Results of 212 consecutive endopyelotomies: an 8-year follow-up. J Urol 149:453–456
11. Robert WW, Cadeddu JA, Micali S, et al. (1998) Ureteral stricture formation after removal of impacted calculi. J Urol 159:723–726
12. Lim DJ, Walker RD III, Ellsworth PI, et al. (1996) Treatment of pediatric urolithiasis between 1984 and 1994. J Urol 156:702–705

Common and Uncommon Complications Related to ESWL

Yasutomo Nasu, Takushi Kurashige, and Hiromi Kumon

Summary. Extracorporeal shock wave lithotripsy (ESWL) is one of the most common urologic procedures performed today. Although it is a minimally invasive procedure, there has been a wide spectrum of injuries to the kidney and adjacent organs associated with ESWL. It is evident that ESWL produces a variety of acute clinical and subclinical complications that may have an effect on long-term blood pressure and renal function. In this chapter, we review the common and uncommon complications related to ESWL based on our multiinstitutional study of 6852 cases treated at Okayama University Hospital and its affiliated hospitals, as well as an intensive literature survey. In our study, we have analyzed the relationship between the incidence of acute symptomatic complications, i.e., post-ESWL fever as a common complication, and renal subcapsular hematoma as an uncommon one, and the kind of shockwave generator used. The overall incidence of post-ESWL fever and subcapsular hematoma was 4.2% and 0.6%, respectively. Electrohydraulic lithotriptors produced a higher incidence of these complications than electromagnetic and piezoelectric lithotriptors. In addition to subcapsular hematoma, we found a variety of other uncommon complications, and the clinical manifestations of these cases are reported along with literature reviews.

Key Words. ESWL, Complication, Subcapsular hematoma, Steinstrasse

Introduction

Extracorporeal shock wave lithotripsy (ESWL) has been established as an effective, safe, and minimally invasive treatment for urolithiasis. However, there has been a wide spectrum of injury to the kidney and adjacent organs associated with ESWL. Problems related to stone fragments and infectious complications may occur even after a technically successful procedure. The long-term effects of

Department of Urology, Okayama University Graduate School of Medicine and Dentistry, 2-5-1 Shikata-cho, Okayama 700-8558, Japan

ESWL on renal function and blood pressure are also important issues to be considered. With regard to these safety issues, a comparison of lithotriptors may be quite difficult, since a variety of lithotriptors with different methods of shockwave generation, power levels, imaging systems, and focal area sizes are being operated by a variety of users in different institutions. In this chapter, we review common and uncommon complications related to ESWL mainly based on our study of 6852 cases treated at Okayama University Hospital and its affiliated hospitals. The incidence of acute symptomatic complications also has been analyzed according to the type of shockwave generators used.

Background of a Multi-Institutional Survey

From 1994 to 1999, 6852 patients (male, 4918; female, 1934; age, 10–91 years; stone size, 1–83 mm) with upper urinary tract stone were treated at Okayama University Hospital and its seven affiliated hospitals (Table 1). All the attending urologists had received the same training course before starting ESWL treatment at each institution. The first lithotriptor employed was the Dornier HM-3 (Dornier Medical Systems, Inc., Wessling, Germany), and we have surveyed six other, different lithotriptors with electrohydraulic, electromagnetic, or piezelectric generators. The number of patients treated with each type of lithotriptor is shown in Table 2. There were no significant differences in patient characteristics among the groups treated with the three different types of shockwave generator (location of stone, kidney 36.4%–39.3%, ureter 60.7%–63.6%; size, >10 mm 42.8%–53.9%; number, multiple stones 14.9%–26.3%). The average number of shock waves applied per patient is shown in Table 1. Overall success rates, defined as complete disappearance or residual stones of less than 4 mm, are 98.5% for the electrohydraulic group, 97.2% for the electromagnetic group, and 96.7% for the piezoelectric group (Table 3). The distribution of patients according to the number of ESWL sessions required for successful treatment with each genera-

TABLE 1. Patient characteristics

No. of patients	6852
Sex	Male 4918, female 1934
Age	10–91 years (median 50 years)
Stone	
Location	Kidney 2529, ureter 4226
Size	1–83 mm (mean 11.4 mm)
Number	Solitary 5029, multiple 1211
ESWL	
No. of sessions	10576 (1.54 sessions/patient)
Average shots of shock waves/patient	
Electrohydraulic	2008 ($n = 841$)
Electromagnetic	2774 ($n = 5502$)
Piezoelectric	3646 ($n = 509$)

TABLE 2. List of lithotriptors and the number of patients treated

Generator	Lithotriptor	No. of patients
Electrohydraulic	HM-3[a]	645
	MPL 9000[a]	196
Electromagnetic	Lithostar[b]	2212
	Lithostar plus[b]	2341
	Modulith SLX[c]	529
	Modulith SL20[c]	420
Piezoelectric	Piezolith 2000[d]	509
Total		6852

[a] Dornier Medical Systems, Inc., Wessling, Germany.
[b] Siemens AG., Munich, Germany.
[c] Storz Medical, Kreuzlingen, Switzerland.
[d] RICHARD WOLF, Knittlingen, Germany.

TABLE 3. Overall success rate and number of sessions employed

	Electrohydraulic ($n = 680$)	Electromagnetic ($n = 4125$)	Piezoelectric ($n = 420$)
Overall success rate (%)[a]	98.5	97.2	96.7
No. of patients (and %)			
1 session	529 (77.8)	2679 (64.9)	271 (64.6)
2 sessions	122 (17.9)	948 (23.0)	63 (14.9)
3 sessions	20 (3.0)	260 (6.3)	29 (6.9)
≥4 sessions	9 (1.3)	238 (5.8)	57 (13.6)
Mean number of sessions	1.25	1.61	2.12

[a] Evaluation 12 weeks after the final ESWL; success is defined as complete disappearance or residual stone of ≤4 mm after ESWL.

tor is also shown in Table 3. More than four sessions were required in 13.6% of patients treated with the piezoelectric lithotriptor.

Common Complications

Common ESWL-related complications result mainly from problems associated with stone fragments, infections associated with the treatment of primary infected stones or infections secondary to ESWL, and direct tissue damage. Pain, fever, and hematuria are the most frequent clinical symptoms which accompany these common complications. Among them, we have selected fever as an easily comparable parameter responsible for acute symptomatic complications.

Post-ESWL Fever

Fever elevation over 38°C on and after post-ESWL day 1, and which is clinically judged as being stone-related, is defined as a positive febrile episode. We have compared the incidence of this post-ESWL fever in relation to the kind of shock-wave generator used. The overall incidence of post-ESWL fever was 4.2% (290/6852). The overall incidence of fever in the treatment of ureteral stone (3.5%) was lower than that in the treatment of renal stone (5.5%), and did not correlate with the size of the ureteral stone (Fig. 1). In cases of renal stone, however, it was evident that the incidence of post-ESWL fever increased in parallel with the size of the renal stone, reaching 28.1% (36/128) for cases with stones of over 40mm. As shown in Fig. 2, electrohydraulic lithotriptors produced the highest (8.76%) and peizoelectric lithotriptors the lowest (0.98%) incidence of post-ESWL fever. There was no significant difference in the incidence of fever between electrohydraulic lithotriptors (HM-3 and MPL 9000).

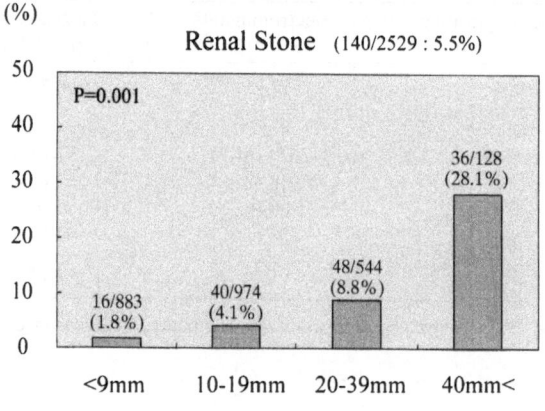

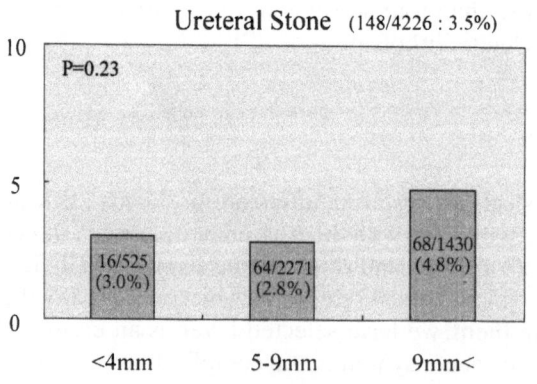

FIG. 1. Incidence of post-ESWL fever according to stone size

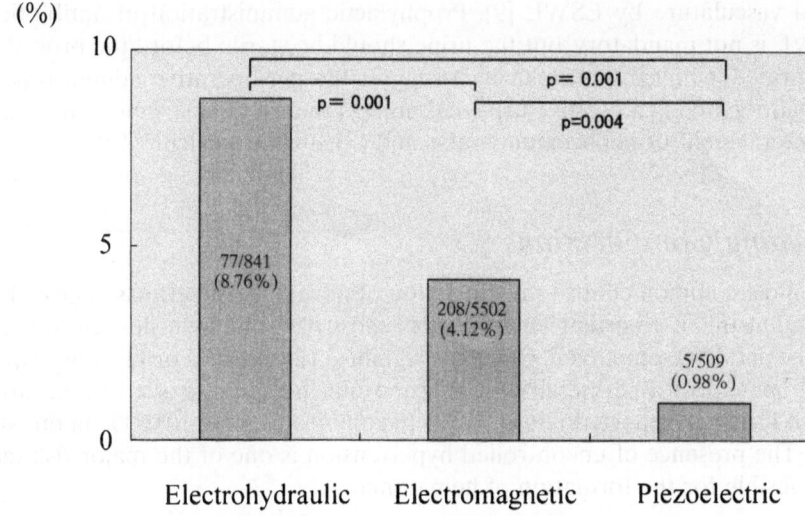

FIG. 2. Incidence of post-ESWL fever according to shockwave generator

Steinstrasse

The most common complications associated with ESWL are problems related to stone fragments. Poor fragmentation and the accumulation of multiple stone fragments causes steinstrasse, resulting in obstruction of the ureter. The risk factors for the formation of steinstrasse have been extensively reviewed: the composition (calcium oxalate monohydrate, calcium phosphate dihydrate, and cystine) and size (over 20–25 mm) of target calculi are major risk factors, and the location of calculi and the type of lithotriptor used are minor ones [1–3]. In our study, the overall incidence of steinstrasse was 2.25% and the average stone size was 19.5 mm (15–65 mm). It has been established that obstructive complications after ESWL can be minimized by pre-ESWL placement of a ureteral stent for a moderate stone burden (aggregate stone diameter more than 25 mm) [4, 5]. We believe that those patients with significant obstruction or infection should be managed with prompt urinary tract decompression by nephrostomy tube placement [6, 7].

Infection

Overall, the reported incidence of sepsis following ESWL is less than 1%, although for staghorn calculi the rate is 2.7% [1, 8]. In our study, the incidence of sepsis was less than 0.1%, but three cases developed serious septic shock. A positive urine culture and urinary obstruction are risk factors of sepsis. The systemic transfer of bacteria is facilitated through the mechanical manipulation of renal vasculature by ESWL [9]. Prophylactic administration of antibiotics for ESWL is not mandatory, but the urine should be sterile before the procedure is performed. Clinical features which suggest the perioperative administration of antibiotics are (1) a positive urine culture, (2) the use of instrumentation such as a ureteral stent or nephrostomy tube, and (3) staghorn calculi [10].

Bleeding Complications

The most common clinical manifestation of adverse renal effects is gross hematuria, but this is transient and occurs in most patients regardless of the energy source and level employed. Clinically significant hematuria or bleeding, with the development of a perinephric or subcapusular hematoma, is a rare occurrence which has been reported in only 0.1% to 0.66% of patients (0.63% in our study) [11]. The presence of uncontrolled hypertension is one of the major risk factors responsible for the formation of hematoma.

Long-Term Complications

Numerous studies document changes in biochemical markers which indicate damage to the nephron. However, there are no published data showing that ESWL produces a significant long-term adverse effect on renal function. A large-scale prospective study is needed to elucidate this most important issue.

The association of ESWL with the onset of de novo hypertension is also a major concern. In animal models, renin levels are elevated following ESWL [12], and it is speculated that renal fibrosis formed by hematoma in turn causes renal compression and decreases perfusion, leading to increased renin release and subsequent hypertension [13, 14]. In 1987, Lingeman and Kulb [15] initially reported that of 243 normotensive patients, 8.2% were hypertensive or on antihypertension medication 1 year after ESWL. Subsequently, several related studies have produced conflicting results [16, 17]. Recent clinical research has focused on identifying patients who may be at increased risk of hypertension. Peschel et al. [18] demonstrated that the incidence of post-ESWL hypertension is related to age. Among patients undergoing ESWL who are over 60, the incidence of post-ESWL hypertension was reported to be 37.5%, which is markedly higher than in the age-matched general population (8.4%).

Uncommon Complications

A variety of uncommon adverse effects and clinical complications associated with ESWL have been reported. In this section, the clinical manifestations of uncommon complications detected in our study are reported (Table 4), along with literature reviews.

TABLE 4. Rare complications

Complication	Generator	Age/sex	Location	Size (mm)	No. of stones	Shots	Sessions	Remarks
Liver injury	Electromagnetic	55/M	R2/Rt	10	Single	3600	1	Cirrhosis with HCC
Ileus	Electromagnetic	53/F	U1/Lt	8	Single	8000	2	Colonic diverticulitis
Ileus	Electromagnetic	53/M	R2/Lt	12	Multiple	4000	1	Cerebral thrombosis Subcapsular hematoma
Arrhythmia	Electromagnetic	74/M	R3/Lt	6	Multiple	8200	2	VPCs
Arrhythmia	Electromagnetic	79/M	R1/Lt	11	Multiple	23100	8	Bradycardia with AF
Cardiac arrest	Electrohydraulic	57/M	U1/Rt	8	Single	2000	5	Vasovagal reflex
Abortion	Electrohydraulic	37/F	U3/Rt	4	Single	2000	1	

R1, kidney or diverticulum; R2, calyx or pelvis; R3, PUJ.
U1, upper ureter; U2, middle ureter; U3, lower ureter.
DIC, disseminated intravascular coagulopathy; HCC, hepatocellular carcinoma; VPCs, ventricular premature contractions; AF, atrial fibrillation.

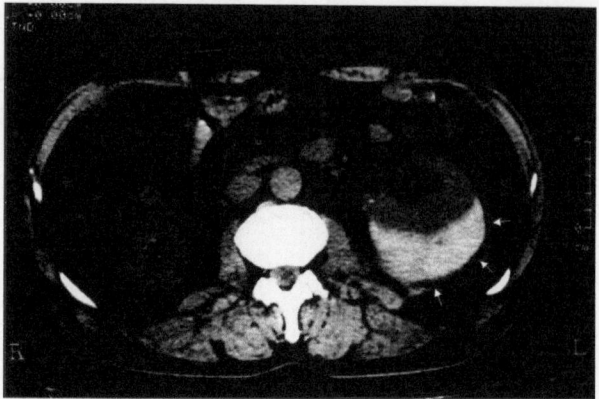

FIG. 3. Subcapsular hematoma. One day after initial ESWL for a left upper ureteral stone, the patient complained of left abdominal pain. A computed tomography (CT) scan revealed subcapsular hematoma formation (*white arrows*). An anticoagulant agent for cerebral thrombosis was discontinued 7 days before ESWL, and no abnormal laboratory data were obtained in pre-ESWL coagulatory tests. The patient was managed conservatively without surgical intervention or transfusion

Damage to Target Organ

An uncommon and critical manifestation of an adverse renal effect is subcapsular or perirenal hematoma. In our study, there were 43 cases (0.6%) of subcapsular or perirenal hematoma, which were diagnosed by (1) routine post-ESWL ultrasound examination, or (2) computed tomography (CT) scan, which was used in cases with indicative symptoms or laboratory abnormalities such as anemia (Fig. 3). No patients received open surgical intervention, but blood transfusion was necessary for one patient who had liver cirrhosis with a subclinical bleeding disorder. We have analyzed the incidence of hematoma according to the type of shockwave generator used (Fig. 4). Although the result is not statistically significant, electrohydraulic lithotriptors produced the highest incidence of hematoma (0.83%) and the peizoelectric lithotriptor lowest (0.2%).

Damage to Adjacent Organs

Adjacent organs susceptible to shock waves are reported to be the liver, lungs, stomach, intestines, and pancreas. Gastric or duodenal erosion, pancreatitis, and mucosal erosion of the colon have been reported, but were minor and transient.

There was one case of liver injury in our series (see Table 4). The patient's underlying condition of liver cirrhosis with hepatocellular carcinoma was diagnosed after ESWL. Pre-ESWL examination did not reveal any bleeding disorder, but subclinical coagulopathy might have been a predisposing factor in this case. Four cases of liver injury have previously been reported in the literature

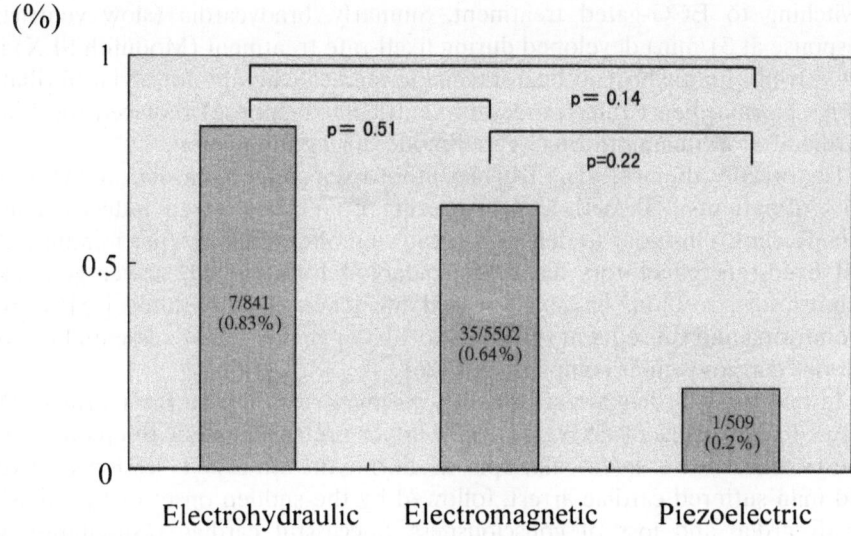

Fig. 4. Incidence of hematoma according to shockwave generator

Table 5. Cases of liver injury after ESWL

Case	Age/sex	Stone location	Predisposing factor	Treatment	References
1	30/F	Rt. kidney	None	Ligation of rt. hepatic artery	Bogdanovic et al. [19]
2	25/M	Rt. upper ureter	None	Embolization	Harada et al. [20]
3	69/M	Rt. kidney	None	Drainage	Meyer and Cass [21]
4	63/F	Rt. kidney	Hypertension	Conservative	Kobayasi et al. [22]
5	55/M	Rt. kidney	Cirrhosis with HCC	Conservative	Present case

(Table 5) [19–22]; three patients had no abnormalities in their coagulating systems, and the remaining one had hypertension.

There were two cases of post-ESWL paralytic ileus, which is a rare gastrointestinal complication. While the three cases found in the literature were presumed to be related to anesthesia [23, 24], our two cases had received no anesthesia. Although a 53-year-old woman had colonic diverticulitis and a 63-year-old man had cerebral thrombosis as underlying diseases, ESWL-related pain (development of hematoma in the latter case) might have been etiological.

Cardiovascular Complications

In our study, there were two cases of symptomatic arrhythmia. A 74-year-old man showed frequent ventricular premature contractions (VPCs) during external fixed-rate treatment (Modulith SLX) and the arrhythmia disappeared by switching to ECG-gated treatment. Similarly, bradycardia (slow ventricular response at 31/min) developed during fixed-rate treatment (Modulith SLX) in a 79-year-old man who had been receiving medical therapy for atrial fibrillation (AF). Normal heart rate (moderate ventricular response) replaced the brady-cardia after switching to ECG-gated mode during the session.

Historically, the prototype Dornier lithotriptor induced cardiac arrhythmia in 80% of patients [25]. With ECG-triggering, ESWL only rarely induces arrhyth-mia. Recently, in order to deliver a greater number of shocks per minute, exter-nal fixed-rate generators have been adapted for use with newer generation lithotriptors, resulting in an increased incidence of arrhythmia [25]. Careful monitoring and subsequent switching to ECG-gated mode are essential to avoid serious cardiovascular complications [26].

In one case, cardiac arrest occurred during a session with the Dornier HM3. After four sessions of ESWL for right upper ureteral stone with epidural anes-thesia without a cardiovascular episode, during the 5th ESWL session, a 54-year-old man suffered cardiac arrest, followed by the sudden onset of hypotension, bradycardia, and loss of consciousness. Successful cardiac resuscitation was carried out immediately. A post-ESWL cardiovascular examination revealed no abnormality, and an intensive investigation of intraoperative medical records indicated that cardiac arrest might be a manifestation of excessive vasovagal reflex. Two cases of cardiac arrest have been reported in the literature, but no evidence was found that the shock waves rather than vagal activation and the action of sedoanalgesia was the cause [25, 27].

Other Uncommon Complications

We experienced one case of abortion after ESWL. An unmarried 37-year-old woman received ESWL for right lower ureteral stone with no knowledge of the possibility of pregnancy. The day after ESWL, abnormal genital bleeding occurred and gynecological examination revealed spontaneous abortion. The potential effects of the extracorporeal application of shock waves on an embryo or fetus have been explored in an animal model [28]. Embryotoxic or teratogenic sequels did not occur when shock waves were focused outside the uterus. Frankenschmidt and Sommerkamp [29] reported a successful use of ESWL during pregnancy, but the use of ESWL during pregnancy is still contraindicated and undoubtedly controversial.

Concomitant Malignancies

Seven cases of malignant disease (0.1%) were diagnosed incidentally during ESWL procedures (Table 6). Among these seven malignancies, four cases were urological cancer (two cases of bladder cancer and two cases of renal cell carci-noma). The literature reviews of concomitant malignances found during ESWL treatment are shown in Table 7 [30–32]. Urologists have relatively frequent opportunities to encounter urogenital malignancy in connection with ESWL based on the surrogate observation that the corrected estimates of the age-

TABLE 6. Summary of concomitant malignancy

Case	Age/sex	Site of malignancy	Stone location	Time of diagnosis	Treatment
1	47/M	Bladder	Lt. ureter (U1)	During ESWL	TUR-Bt
2	53/M	Bladder	Lt. ureter (U2)	Before ESWL	TUR-Bt
3	58/M	Rt. kidney	Rt. kidney (R2)	7 days after ESWL	Nephrectomy
4	68/M	Lt. kidney	Lt. kidney (R2)	2 months after ESWL	Nephrectomy
5	75/F	Pancreas	Lt. kidney (R3)	3 days after ESWL	Conservative
6	54/M	Liver	Rt. kidney (R1)	1 day after ESWL, with renal subcapsular hematoma	Conservative
7	55/M	Liver	Rt. kidney (R1)	1 day after ESWL, with liver injury	Conservative

TUR-Bt, transurethral resection of bladder tumor.

TABLE 7. Literature review of concomitant malignancy found in ESWL

References	No. patients	Nonurogenital neoplasm (%)	Urogenital neoplasm (%)	Kidney (%)	Renal pelvis/ureter (%)	Bladder (%)	Remarks
Yokoyama et al. [30]	2686	11 (0.4)	14 (0.52)	5 (0.19)	3 (0.11)	4 (0.15)	Prostate 1, penis 1
Kamihara et al. [31]	4418	NA	11 (0.25)	4 (0.09)	2 (0.05)	5 (0.11)	
Kitamura et al. [32]	564	2 (0.35)	4 (0.71)	1 (0.18)	1 (0.18)	2 (0.35)	
Present Study	6852	3 (0.04)	4 (0.06)	2 (0.03)	0	2 (0.03)	

Corrected estimates of age-standardized rate per 100000 population in Japan: kidney, 7.0; bladder, 10.7.
NA, not applicable.

standardized rates of bladder cancer and renal cell carcinoma in Japan are 10.7 (0.01%) and 7.0 (0.007%) per 100000, respectively. To prove this hypothesis, further prospective studies are needed for a comparison with a control group of patients visiting urologic clinics.

We experienced one case of renal cancer (case 4), which showed progressive and disseminated growth with poor prognosis shortly after ESWL. Briefly, a 68-year-old man with left renal stone received six sessions of ESWL for 4 months, and a CT scan taken 2 months after the final session revealed a left renal mass with diffuse extension to surrounding tissue and paraaortic mass formation. (Fig. 5). Radical surgery was indicated, but because of severe adhesion to surrounding tissues, simple nephrectomy, rather than radical nephrectomy and paraaortic lymph node dissection, was performed. The patient died 2 months after surgery owing to rapid and disseminated disease progression with multiple lymph node metastases and lung metastases. A pre-ESWL CT indicated the possible existence of a renal tumor when investigated and analyzed retrospectively (Fig. 5). The biological effects of shock waves on malignant tumors vary from cytotoxic effects to an accelerating effect on metastases [33, 34]. Oosterhof et al. [34]

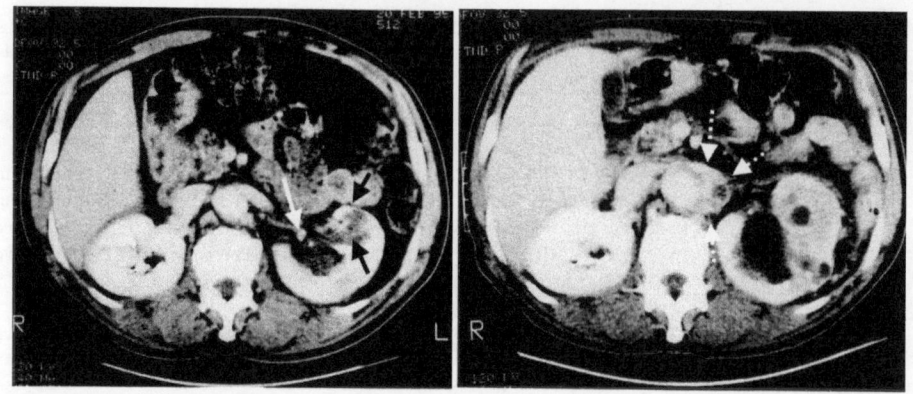

a   b

FIG. 5. Enhanced CT scans. **a** A pre-ESWL CT scan showing a small renal stone (*white arrow*) with hydronephrosis. A low-density area can be seen in the right kidney (*black arrow*). **b** CT scan taken 2 months later after six sessions of ESWL for 4 months, showing a right renal mass extending extracapsularly. The abdominal aorta is surrounded by a mixed density mass suspiciously like lymph node metastasis (*dotted white arrow*)

investigated the hypothesis that exposure of a solid tumor to high-energy shock waves could lead to an increase of metastases in an animal model, and indicated that the metastatic spread of tumors may be enhanced by shockwave exposure when the existing tumor has a high metastatic potential. In spite of the lack of supportive evidence and similar clinical reports, this rare case warrants clinical interest, as does the hypothesis that exposure of the preexisting tumor to shock waves may enhance tumor growth and metastatic potential in some limited circumstances.

Conclusion

ESWL will remain the first choice of treatment modality for upper urinary tract calculi, and our results have reconfirmed its relative safety. In spite of small percentages, a definitive number of critical complications and incidentally diagnosed malignant diseases were present. Urologists using this important technology should be aware that shock waves do not pass harmlessly through the body. Fuchs [35] has indicated that most ESWL complications are user-induced and fall into the basic categories of inappropriate indication for ESWL, imprudent use of the shockwave energy, insufficient follow-up, or unfamiliarity with endourological auxiliary procedures. In order to reduce the incidence and degree of complications, urologists must be knowledgeable about its common and uncommon complications and risk factors. Future clinical research may focus on how to make use of ESWL more efficiently and cost-effectively. However, in addition, continued concern and efforts to reach a better understanding of the effects of shock waves on living tissue remain important in order to enhance the safety profile of ESWL. Renal dysfunction and hypertension are areas in which further examination is necessary. Carefully planned clinical trials and experimental studies are still needed to minimize ESWL-associated complications and elucidate the long-term effects on renal function and hypertension.

References

1. Dretler SP (1988) Stone fragility—a new therapeutic distinction. J Urol 139: 1124–1127
2. American Urological Association (1986) Report of the American Urological Association ad hoc committee to study the safety and efficacy of combined technology of percutaneous lithotripsy and non-invasive lithotripsy. Baltimore
3. Pittomvils G, Vandeursen H, Wevers M, Lafaut JP, De Ridder D, De Meester P, Boving R, Baert L (1994) The influence of internal stone structure upon the fracture behaviour of urinary calculi. Ultrasound Med Bio 20:803–810
4. Libby JM, Meacham RB, Griffith DP (1988) The role of silicone ureteral stents in extracorporeal shock wave lithotripsy of large renal calculi. J Urol 139:15–17
5. Al-Awadi KA, Abdul Halim H, Kehinde EO, Al-Tawheed A (1999) Steinstrasse. A comparison of incidence with and without J-stenting and the effect of J–stenting on subsequent management BJU Int 84:618–621
6. Sigman M, Laudone V, Jenkins AD (1988) Ureteral meatotomy as a treatment of steinstrasse following extracorporeal shock wave lithotripsy. J Endourol 2:41
7. Joshi HB, Obadeyi OO, Rao PN (1999) A comparative analysis of nephrostomy, JJ stent and urgent in situ extracorporeal shock wave lithotripsy for obstructing ureteric stones. BJU Int 84:264–269
8. Lam HS, Lingeman JE, Barron M, Newman DM, Mosbaugh PG, Steele RE, Knapp PM, Scott JW, Nyhuis A, Woods JR (1992) Staghorn calculi: analysis of treatment results between initial percutaneous nephrostolithotomy and extracorporeal shock wave lithotripsy monotherapy with reference to surface area. J Urol 147:1219
9 Muller-Mattheis VGO, Schmale D, Seewald M, Rosin H, Ackermann R (1991) Bacteremia during extracorporeal shock wave lithotripsy of renal calculi. J Urol 146:733–736
10. Newmark JR, Wong MYC, Lingemar JE (1996) Complications. In: Smith AD (ed) Smith's textbook of endourology. Quality Medical Publishing, St. Louis, pp 680–693
11. Knapp PM, Kulb TB, Lingeman JE, Newman DM, Mertz JH, Mosbaugh PG, Steele RE (1988) Extracorporeal shock wave lithotripsy-induced perirenal hematomas. J Urol 139:700–703
12. Neal DE, Harmon E, Hlavinka T (1991) Effects of multiple sequential extracorporeal shock wave treatments on renal function: a primate model. J Endourol 5:217
13. Karlsen SJ, Berg KJ (1992) Changes in renal function after extracorporeal shock wave lithotripsy in patients with solitary functioning kidneys: long-term follow up. J Endourol 6:205
14. Lemann J, Taylor AJ, Collier BD, Lipchik EO (1991) Kidney hematoma due to extracorporeal shock wave lithotripsy causing transient renin-mediated hypertension. J Urol 145:1238–1241
15. Lingeman JE, Kulb TB (1987) Hypertension following extracorporeal shock wave lithotripsy. J Urol 137:142A
16. Claro J de A, Lima ML, Ferreira U, Rodrigues Netto N Jr (1993) Blood pressure changes after extracorporeal shock wave lithotripsy in normotensive patients. J Urol 150:1765–1767

17. Yokoyama M, Shoji F, Yanagisawa R, Kanemura M, Kitahara K, Takahasi S, Kawai K, Oda H, Osaka M, Handa H (1992) Blood pressure changes following extracorporeal shock wave lithotripsy for urolithiasis. J Urol 147:553–558

18. Peschel R, Janetschek G, Frauscher F, Hofle G, Bartsch G (1997) Does ESWL induce hypertension in the elderly. J Urol 157:272 (abstract)

19. Bogdanovic J, Mirkovic M, Idjuski S, Popov M, Marusic G, Stojkov J (1999) Liver injury related to extracorporeal shock wave lithotripsy in a quadriplegic patient. BJU Int 83:718–719

20. Harada H, Taniguchi K, Nantani M, Matsumoto T, Nonomura K, Koyanagi T (1994) Hepatic subcapsular hematoma after ESWL for a renal stone: a case report. Jpn J Endourol ESWL 7:233–235

21. Meyer JJ, Cass AS (1995) Subcapsular hematoma of the liver after renal extracorporeal shock wave lithotripsy. J Urol 154:516–517

22. Kobayashi K, Ishizuka E, Iwasaki A, Saito R (1998) Subcapsular hematoma of the liver after extracorporeal shock wave lithotripsy. Jpn J Urol 89:445–448

23. Ono Y, Sahashi M, Watanabe J, Yamada S, Kamihira O, Hirabayashi S, Nakano Y, Miyake K, Ohshima S (1991) Extracorporeal shock wave lithotripsy monotherapy in the treatment of staghorn calculi. Jpn J Urol 82:433–438

24. Jenkins AD, Gillenwater JY (1988) Extracorporeal shock wave lithotripsy in the prone position: treatment of stones in the distal ureter or anomalous kidney. J Urol 139: 911–915

25. Zeng ZR, Lindstedt E, Roijer A, Olsson SB (1993) Arrhythmia during extracorporeal shock wave lithotripsy. Br J Urol 71:6–10

26. Ganem JP, Carson CC (1998) Cardiac arrhythmias with external fixed-rate signal generators in shock wave lithotripsy with the Medstone lithotripter. Urology 51: 548–552

27. Sofras F, Karayannis A, Kostakopoulos A, Delakas D, Kastriotis J, Dimopoulos C (1988) Methodology, results and complications in 2000 extracorporeal shock wave lithotripsy procedures. Br J Urol 61:9–13

28. Frankenschmidt A, Heisler M (1998) Fetotoxicity and teratogenesis of SWL treatment in the rabbit. J Endourol 12:15–21

29. Frankenschmidt A, Sommerkamp H (1998) Shock wave lithotripsy during pregnancy: a successful clinical experiment. J Urol 159:501–502

30. Yokoyama M, Kanemura M, Kitahara K (1994) C-existence of malignant neoplasms and stones in the upper urinary tract—a hidden risk during ESWL treatment. Jpn J Endourol ESWL 7:53–56

31. Kamihara O, Ohshima S, Ono Y (1996) ESWL treatment and the detection of urological neoplasm. Jpn J Endourol ESWL 9:105–108

32. Kitamura H, Aoki M, Wada H (1997) Malignant neoplasm incidentally found in ESWL treatment. Jpn J Endourol ESWL 10:57–59

33. Hoshi S, Orikasa S, Suzuki K, Saitoh T, Takahashi T, Yoshikawa K, Kuwahara M, Nose M (1995) High-energy underwater shock wave treatment for internal iliac muscle metastasis of prostatic cancer: a first clinical trial. Jpn J Cancer Res 86:424–428

34. Oosterhof GO, Cornel EB, Smits GA, Debruyne FM, Schalken JA (1996) The influence of high-energy shock waves on the development of metastases. Ultrasound Med Biol 22:339–344

35. Fuchs JG (1994) Renal stones: extracorporeal shock wave lothotripsy. In: Krane RJ, Siroky MB, Fitzpatrick JM (eds) Clinical urology. Lippincott, Philadelphia, pp 289–302

Complications of Urolithiasis Treatment (PNL)

TAIJI NISHIMURA

Summary. Percutaneous nephrolithotomy (PNL) and its related procedures still have important roles in endourology, e.g., for patients with staghorn calculi, low caliceal stones, ESWL-resistant calculi, and percutaneous endopyelotomy. Therefore, it is worth reviewing the possible complications with PNL treatment. Even nowadays, with our advanced techniques, common complications such as hemorrhage or infection, and rare complications such as the puncture of adjacent organs are reported. This chapter reviews the complications which can occur with PNL, with the emphasis on recent reports. The case of hemorrhage requiring blood transfusion has not been described in recent papers, but indications for angiography and embolization upon profuse bleeding have been described, and are quoted here. Experienced urologists should be grateful to authors who report rare cases of complications, because this information may be used to avoid a potentially devastating complication in the future. In addition, well-known methods to deal with hemostasis and the prevention of postoperative urinary tract infection will be beneficial for beginners, so that they will not be excessively worried by profuse bleeding, and will know how to prevent urosepsis.

Key Words. Percutaneous nephrolithotomys, Percutaneous nephrostomy, Urolithiasis

Introduction

Percutaneous nephrolithotomy (PNL) and its related procedures still have important roles in endourology, e.g., for patients with staghorn calculi, low caliceal stones, ESWL-resistant calculi, and percutaneous endopyelotomy. Therefore, it is worth reviewing the possible complications with PNL treatment.

Department of Urology. Nippon Medical School, 1-1-5 Sendagi, Bunkyo-ku, Tokyo 113-8603, Japan

TABLE 1. Complications with PNL

Complication	Incidence (%)			
	Tanahashi et al. [1]	Roth and Beekmann [2]	Tsuboi et al. [3]	Shishido et al. [4]
Number of cases	522	Review	243	103
Year published	1987	1988	1989	1990
Renal hemorrhage[a]	5.4	2–11	12.8	8.8
UPJ and ureteral stenosis	0.6	0.1–0.8	0.4	1.9
Bowel injury	0.0	0.1	0.0	0.0
Pneumothorax, hemothorax	0.2	0.1–3.0	0.0	0.0
Fever (>38°C), sepsis	9.4	0.2–2.6	ND	8.8
Myocardial infarction	0.0	0.1–0.4	0.4	0.0

[a] Hemorrhage requiring blood transfusion.
UPJ, ureteropehic junction; ND, no data.

The incidence of complications with PNL reported during 1987–1990 is shown in Table 1 [1–4]. Such complications, especially those concerning injury to adjacent organs, are not well reported in the Japanese literature, but are extensively described in the English literature [2, 5–7]. Even nowadays, with advanced techniques, rare complications are reported from other countries, possibly because of differences in body shape, most likely due to marked obesity. Japanese urologists can benefit from this information because they may need to avoid potentially devastating complications in the future. This review of complications with PNL concentrates on recent reports.

Anesthesia

In epidural anesthesia, which is the most popular method of anesthesia for PNL, the duration of anesthesia must be 3h or less in the young, and 2h or less in elderly patients in order to prevent dyspnea.

Watanabe et al. [8] reported a case of sudden cardiac arrest at the beginning of PNL without hemorrhage. They concluded that the cause of this cardiac arrest might have been the suppression of respiration due to inadvertent and inappropriate expansion of the area of epidural anesthesia and/or vagus reflex caused by stimulation due to PNL procedures which could not be blocked by epidural anesthesia. Although the patient was resuscitated with epinephrine, calcium chloride, and sodium bicarbonate, these authors recommend general anesthesia with intubation because of the ease of resuscitation in a prone position. Morbidly obese patients undergoing PNL may be more likely to have respiratory complications intraoperatively and postoperatively, and maintaining an airway in these patients when they are in the prone position may be particularly difficult without intubation.

Complications During Nephrostomy Procedures

Allergic Reaction to Contrast Medium

An allergic reaction to the contrast medium is definitely one possible complication with PNL. The management of patients with a history of allergic reaction using steroids and antihistamine before using any contrast medium is similar to the standard method [5].

Air Embolism

In a case reported by Cadeddu et al. [9], the injection of 10 cc of air was repeated because of a failure to pass the guide wire to the renal pelvis, and the second injection caused sudden oxygen desaturation, bradycardia, and hypotension due to air embolism. The patient was resuscitated by mechanical ventilation, chest compression, and the administration of atropine, epinephrine, and phenylephrine. However, a puncture with the use of air should be replaced by an ultrasound-guided puncture.

Hemorrhage

Excessive bleeding can occur during any phase of PNL, e.g., needle passage, tract dilatation, nephrolithotomy, or the postoperative period. The incidence of blood loss in PNL which was severe enough to necessitate blood transfusion, and which appeared in the literature published in the late 1980s, was 1% to 11% [2]. With advances in the technique of renal puncture, the current incidence would be expected to be lower than in the past. However, the incidences that have appeared in recent papers were higher, i.e., 20% and 23% [10, 11]. Davidoff and Bellman [10] reported that balloon tract dilators led to less renal hemorrhage and lower transfusion rates compared with Amplatz dilatation. Stoller et al. [11] reported that multiple punctures and/or renal pelvic perforation was associated with a two-fold greater blood loss, while half of the expected blood loss occurred in patients with a preexisting nephrostomy tract. Anemia [11] and coagulopathic conditions are significant risk factors influencing the likelihood of a marked hemorrhage or a blood transfusion. The incidence of hemorrhage in PNL is higher than that in percutaneous nephrostomy (PCN) because of the site-specific nature, larger caliber nephrostomy tract, and endoscopic procedures in the former. However, PCN is often performed as an emergency procedure, and consequently the mortality rate in 1207 PCNs reported by Stable [12] in 1982, when the techniques and equipment for PCN were not as advanced as those available today, was as high as 0.2%. However, all the patients who died had either a specific coagulation disorder or coagulopathy associated with advanced uremia. Kessaris et al. [13] reported that even if the patient has a normal partial thromboplastin time, prothrombin time, and platelet count preoperatively, a coagulopathic condition may be present, and therefore the operation should not proceed if the patient has profuse bleeding immediately after needle insertion. Mahaffey et al. [14] reported that nephrostomy tubes must be placed by urologists and not by interventional radiologists because the decision to place a nephrostomy tube is usually made under the direction of a urologist, and the urologist will ultimately direct long-term follow-up, can assess when tubes should be replaced, and has the most knowledge about determining the entry site into the collecting system if used for endourological procedures. They also report that their series demonstrated that the placement of percutaneous nephrostomy could be performed with morbidity rates similar to those of the best reports documented by radiologists. Bleeding during the procedure of making the nephrostomy is most often venous, as in most other phases of PNL, and not profuse enough to be regarded as a complication. Even profuse bleeding due to arterial injury such as renal segmental artery injury usually stops with pressure using a dilator, working sheath, or endoscope as long as the bleeding site is located in the nephrostomy tract. The placement of a Kaye tamponade balloon catheter [15] (Fig. 1) may be useful if pressure with the aforementioned instruments does not work. However, if the bleeding site is located somewhere other than the nephrostomy tract, such as in the urothelium of the pelvis or the calix, or in the peripelvic area preceded by false passage of the dilator due to inappropriate location of the tip of the guide wire, clamping of the nephrostomy tube for 2–4h may be required to stop the bleeding. Second-stage PNL is one possible choice to minimize the complication of profuse bleeding. Larger arteries, such as a major branch of the renal artery, or even the inferior vena cava or portal vein [7], may be punctured, especially in patients with an unusual body shape such as marked kyphosis or scoliosis, morbid obesity or thinness, in uncooperative patients with local anesthesia, and with operators who are beginners. Those unfavorable conditions are also risk factors in injuring the urinary tract and adjacent organs. Cowan et al. [16] recently reported a rare case of puncturing a major branch of the right renal artery which was treated by percutaneous transrenal embolization. The injury of blood vessels during puncture and dilatation may cause bleeding upon removal of the nephrostomy and arteriovenous fistula or pseudoaneurysm, as considered in the following sections.

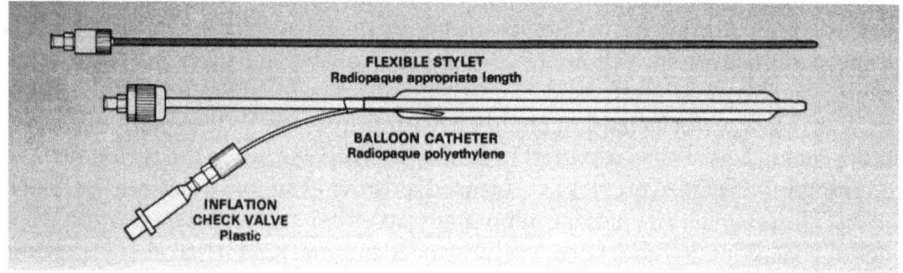

Fɪɢ. 1. Kaye tamponade balloon

FIG. 2. Resin-injected cast of renal blood vessels. View from anterior renal surface to posterior renal surface (*upper*) and view from the outer convex border to renal hilum (*lower*)

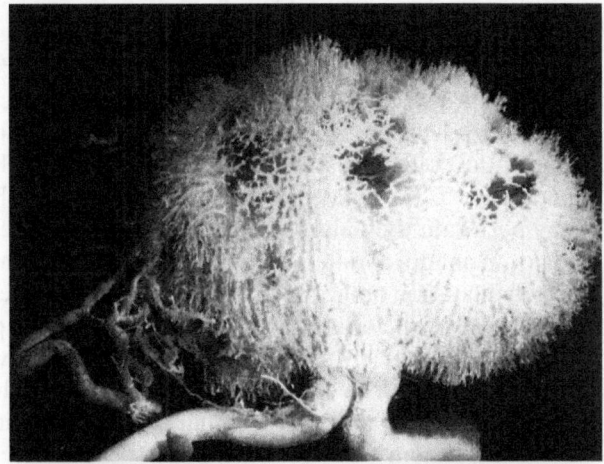

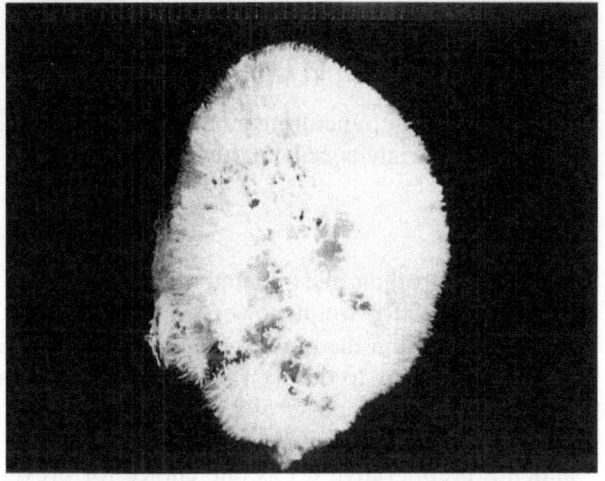

To prevent hemorrhage, most text books mention that ultrasound-guided puncture should be performed with a posterolateral infracostal approach close to Brodel's avascular plane and via the fornix of a calyx to prevent injuring the interlobar and segmental arteries. This is absolutely true, but in the way that the needle of a sextant biopsy of the prostate may or may not hit a cancer lesion, even when the operator performs the procedure as mentioned in the textbook, the needle may or may not hit an interlobar or segmental artery because the kidney has an abundance of blood vessels, as shown by resin-injected casts of the rabbit kidney (Fig. 2) [17]. However, the operator should not be excessively worried about hemorrhage in PNL as long as they are aware of the aforementioned information about hemostasis.

Urinary Tract Injury

Ureteral injuries associated with PNL occur in 0.1% to 1.9% of cases (see Table 1). Puncture of the urinary tract is unlikely to occur as long as the puncturing needle is advanced using an ultrasound guide. Also, the needle should be fixed against the collecting system until the injection of the dye and the passage of the guide wire to the collecting system are finished, otherwise, the tip of the needle may perforate the pelvis or injure the renal parenchym and the guide wire may go to an inappropriate position. Even after passage of the guide wire to the ureter, dilatation of the nephrostomy tract can also cause perforation of the pelvis if insertion of the dilator is too deep to touch and penetrate the pelvic wall and it goes in a relatively straight line instead of a curved line along with the guide wire to the ureter. To avoid this injury, the dilator should be inserted just beyond the renal calix so that the maximal-diameter portion of each dilator enters the collecting system.

Puncture of Adjacent Organs

The incidence of puncturing adjacent organs in PNL is higher than that in PCN because of the site-specific nature of the former.

Colon

The adjacent organ most commonly injured is the colon. Colonic injury during PNL occurs with a frequency of 0.2%–0.5% [18]. Colon injury may occur if the colon is located in the path of the nephrostomy tract in the prone position. This condition is likely to occur in patients with a megacolon, malpositioned kidney, colon located in a posterolateral or retrorenal position, marked scoliosis or kyphosis, or morbid obesity or thinness, and is more common on the left. In these patients, preoperative CT is one choice for preventing colon injury. The injury is usually recognized on the postprocedure nephrostogram, which will show contrast material in the colon [5]. Colonic injury should also be suspected postoperatively in patients who experience unexplained fever, prolonged ileus, unexplained leukocytosis, rectal bleeding, evidence of peritoneal inflammation, or fecal/pneumouria [18]. Air in the renal collecting system on plain film is also a sign of colonic–calyceal fistula; however, one should keep in mind that negative pressure developing within the kidney due to hiccups also causes pneumocalyx [19].

If the perforation is extraperitoneal, the problem is simply managed by pulling the nephrostomy tube posteriorly until its tip is in the colon, with placement of a retrograde stent to drain urine. The treatment for a colon injury is the same even in PNL for renal stones in patients who have had sigmoid conduit urinary diversion [18]. However, if intraperitoneal extravasation of contrast material is present, a laparotomy and repair of the bowel is recommended to avoid peritonitis [5]. Of 14 cases of colonic injury associated with PNL reported in the literature to date,

11 were managed conservatively and three required surgical intervention because of peritonitis, pneumoperitoneum, or hemorrhage [18, 20].

Duodenum

Duodenal injuries occur during percutaneous access secondary to guide-wire or dilator perforation through the renal pelvis and into the duodenum, or slipping of the dilator medially over the renal capsule [21]. In either situation, all recently reported cases with duodenal injury were managed conservatively with duodenal drainage, ureteral stent, and parenteral nutrition [22].

Liver

Puncture of the liver does not cause noticeable complications. Roth and Beckmann [2] cited the fact that in percutaneous biliary drainage the catheter is routinely inserted through the liver as evidence of the safety of puncturing the liver.

Spleen

Puncture of the spleen necessitates repair or even splenectomy in some instances. Recently, Kondas et al. [23] reported a case of splenectomy for subcapsular hematoma caused by PNL for left staghorn stone through the 11th–12th rib intercostal approach. In patients with splenomegaly, a more posterior approach should be chosen for the nephrostomy puncture to avoid puncturing the spleen. Beale et al. [24] reported success with left nephrostomy for PNL under CT guidance using a more posterior approach than would be possible with ultrasonography even in patients with massive splenomegaly. Hopper and Yakes [25] recommend puncturing with maximal expiration to prevent spleen injury when the 11th–12th posterior intercostal approach is used for percutaneous access to the upper poles of the kidney. Reinberg et al. [26] reported a case with splenic abscess which was caused by percutaneous nephrostomy tube placement through the spleen with infection. In this case, they pointed out that splenic perforation producing severe hemorrhage did not occur; however, perforation by the guide wire permitted the passage of *Proteus*-infected urine into the spleen. Splenic abscess should be considered in a patient in whom sepsis or left lower pulmonary effusion develops after percutaneous manipulation of the kidney. The treatment of choice for splenic abscess is percutaneous drainage or splenectomy [26].

Gall Bladder

Biliary peritonitis is an uncommon complication of percutaneous approaches, and in a report of over 8000 PNL procedures, this particular complication was not listed [27]. However, if the needle has punctured the common bile duct or gall bladder, which is suggested by aspiration of greenish fluid, it may cause bile leakage followed by biliary peritonitis within 12–48h after the procedure. Puncture of the gall bladder in PCN or PNL caused biliary peritonitis with abdominal pain, distension and tenderness, in three recently reported cases [27–29].

Puncture of Pleura and Lung

In a supracostal approach, a pleurotomy occurs in approximately 12% of cases, and this complication is more commonly associated with a hydrothorax than a pneumothorax after PNL, as discussed in the following section [5].

Complications During Nephrolithotomy

Bleeding

Maneuvers in disintegrating stones using various machines may cause bleeding due to false passage or perforation of the collecting system into the renal parenchyma [7]. Acute loss of the nephrostomy tract is also one of the causes of bleeding in this phase, as well as in the puncturing and dilatation phase in PNL.

Venous bleeding is suspected when the visual field is clear while the irrigation fluid is flowing but is quickly obscured by dark blood when the irrigation is slowed or stopped. Arterial bleeding or major venous bleeding obscures the field even with gravity irrigation [3], and irrigation with pressure is required to obtain a good view. The method of overcoming bleeding is described in the previous section and the following section; however, it may be wise to stop the procedure upon profuse bleeding, leave the nephrostomy, and delay stone removal for 3–7 days to allow the nephrostomy tract to mature.

Injury of the Urinary Tract

Injury of the urinary tract can occur as a result of endoscopic maneuvers. For further information, see the section on late complications.

Complications due to Irrigation Fluid

Hydrothorax and Hydroabdomen

Hemothorax, or hydrothorax, has been reported in 0.1%–3% of patients [1, 2, 7] with the use of intercostal (11th intercostal space) puncture. The common etiological factor is the failure to maintain a sheath in the track during the endoscopic manipulations. To prevent this, the working sheath should be kept in place during endoscopy whenever an 11th intercostal space puncture is performed. Nephrostomies below the 12th rib are associated with an incidence of pleuropulmonary complications of only 1% [7].

A renopleural fistula can be healed by a chest tube and ureteral stent [30]. Hydrothorax and hydroabdomen also tend to occur when a small-caliber 11F sheath and 7F endoscope are used with high-pressure irrigation and without free egress of fluid in children. Pugach et al. [31] recommended monitoring pulmonary compromise and the flank and chest for signs of fluid extravasation during PCNL in children.

A perforation of the collecting system can occur at any time during stone removal, and may cause extravasation of the irrigating fluid into the peritoneal cavity, retroperitoneum, or intravascular space.

Hypothermia

Roberts et al. [32] reported a mean drop of core body temperature of 2°C in PNL, which may cause hypoxia, ischemic injury, or myocardial ischemia, especially in patients with preexisting cardiopulmoanry disease.

Complications Immediately or After Nephrolithotomy

Infection

Infection or sepsis can occur even with a simple nephrostomy, and it is commonplace for the patient to have a fever spike in the evening after PNL [5]. Septic shock has been reported in 0.2%–2.6% of patients treated with PNL [2]. Charton et al. [33] studied the percentage of postoperative urinary tract infection in 107 patients without infection preoperatively in the absence of prophylactic antibiotics, and found that 37 patients (35%) suffered a postoperative urinary tract infection. Therefore, these authors recommend short-term antibiotic prophylaxis.

The presence of bacteria in the urinary tract or in a stone, plus high pressure in the urinary tract caused by obstruction, or the injection of dye or irrigation fluid, may cause septic shock. There may be liver dysfunction, which causes impairment of phagocytosis or detoxification of endotoxins. Measures to prevent septic shock include preoperative administration of antibiotics, and minimizing the pressure in the urinary tract during procedures using the working sheath [34]. However, despite sterilization of the urine with appropriate antibiotic therapy preoperatively, up to 30% of patients who have undergone PNL have bacteriuria. Takeuchi et al. [35] studied fever attacks and their causative factors in PNL and found that fevers were significantly higher and more frequent in cases with infected urinary stones than in those with sterile stones. However, prophylactic administration of antibiotics did not lower the fever or the frequency of fever attacks. They also found that fever was frequent with infected stones such as struvite, but fever was also noted with oxalate calcium stones. This was in agreement with the author's findings that bacteria were recovered even from oxalate calcium stones [36]. Rao et al. [37] reported that the presence of preoperative endotoxemia, bacteriuria, and pyuria are important predictors of postoperative septic shock. Clayman et al. [5] recommend the postponement of further procedures for several days if the urine obtained upon puncture is cloudy or purulent.

Figure 3 shows a summary of the clinical course of a 55-year-old woman with left staghorn calculi who had PNL four times, followed by sepsis and disseminated intravascular coagulation (DIC) which was cured by the administration of

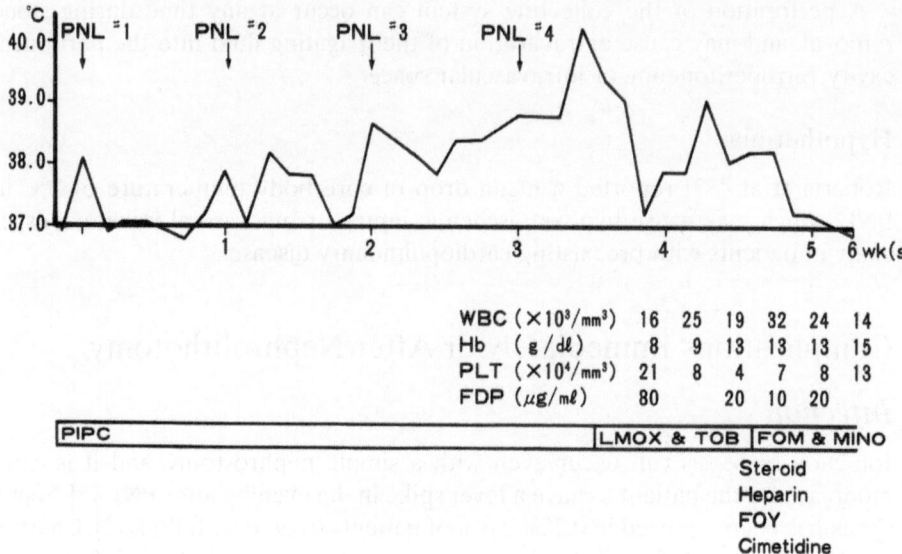

FIG. 3. Summary of the clinical course of a 55-year-old woman with left staghorn calculi who developed sepsis and disseminated intravascular coagulation

TABLE 2. Methods of preventing sepsis

Preoperative administration of antibiotics
Minimize pressure of urinary tract during procedures using working sheath
Postpone further procedure for several days if urine obtained upon puncture is cloudy or purulent

antibiotics, steroids, heparin, gabexate mesilate, cimetidine, and platelets for 3 weeks after the last PNL.

Methods of preventing urinary tract infection or sepsis are summarized in Table 2.

Hemorrhage

An increase in blood pressure after the operation may cause postoperative bleeding, as can occur in transurethral resection of the prostate. Lacerated blood vessels closed by a clot may start to bleed again in the event of increased blood pressure. If the bleeding is profuse, immediate clamping of the nephrostomy is mandatory to save the patient's life, followed by an appropriate treatment for hemostasis, as described below. Arteriovenous fistula or pseudoaneurysma is likely to be another cause of postoperative bleeding during this period. If a lacerated artery leaks into a vein or parenchyma of hilar areolar tissue, it causes an arteriovenous fistula or pseudoaneurysm, respectively [13]. Sacha and Szewczyk

TABLE 3. Summary of cases with profuse hemorrhage requiring angiography and embolization PNL or percutaneous renal surgery

	Incidence	
	---	---
	Kessaris et al. [13]	Sacha and Szewczyk [38]
Year published	1995	1996
Total number of cases	2200	3080
No. of profuse hemorrhages (%)	17 (0.8)	10 (0.3)
Cause of hemorrhage		
AVF (%)	7 (0.32)	4 (0.13)
Pseudoaneurysm (%)	4 (0.18)	2 (0.06)
AVF and pseudoaneurysm (%)	2 (0.09)	
Lacerated renal vessels (%)	2 (0.09)	
Undetermined	2 (0.09)	4 (0.13)

AVF, arteriovenous fistula.

[38] and Kessaris et al. [13] reported the incidence of cases requiring angiography and embolization for significant bleeding uncontrolled by the usual measures, such as clamping of the nephrostomy tube or the use of a balloon tamponade catheter, as 0.3% and 0.8%, respectively (Table 3). In 1995, Kessaris et al. [13] reported that 17 (0.8%) of 2200 percutaneous renal operations required angiography and embolization for significant bleeding, and of these 17 patients, 16 were stone-related procedures. These 17 patients had the following complications: 7 with arteriovenous fistula (0.32%; 7 of 2200); 4 with pseudoaneurysms (0.18%); 2 with arteriovenous fistula and pseudoaneurysm (0.09%); 2 with lacerated renal vessels (0.09%); 2 other cases in which it was not possible to determine the cause.

In 1996, Sacha and Szewczyk [38] described ten patients with massive hemorrhage in 3080 PNL cases; these consisted of 4 arteriovenous fistulae (0.13%; 4 of 3080), 2 aneurysms (0.06%), and 4 other cases in which they were not able to determine the cause. They reported that all arteriovenous fistulae appeared in the kidney's lower pole, and that they punctured and dilated to gain access to the renal pelvis, while they thought sonotrode action might be the cause of aneurysms in the middle part of the kidney in one case.

Hemostasis for arteriovenous fistula and pseudoaneurysm can be performed by angiography and embolization, but nephrectomy is indicated if this is unsuccessful. Sacha and Szewczyk [38] performed a nephrectomy in one patient who developed massive bleeding on the 15th day after PNL, which later became worse. They were unable to find a definite bleeding point.

Kessaris et al. [13] recommend angiography and embolization under the three following conditions: (1) in the immediate postoperative period when clamping of the nephrostomy tube and a tamponade balloon catheter fail to control the hemorrhage (24% of their series); (2) in the early postoperative period (2–7 days)

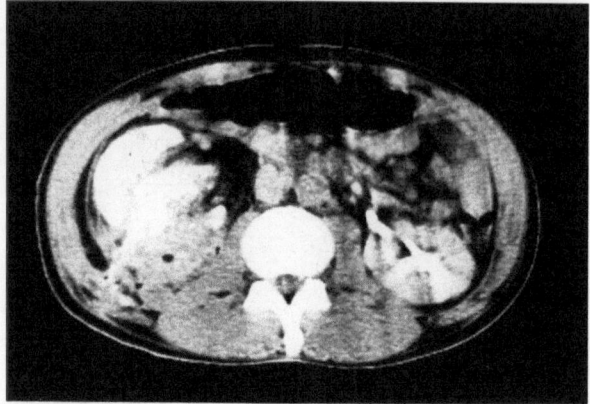

Fig. 4. CT of a perirenal hematoma after PNL for right complete staghorn calculi

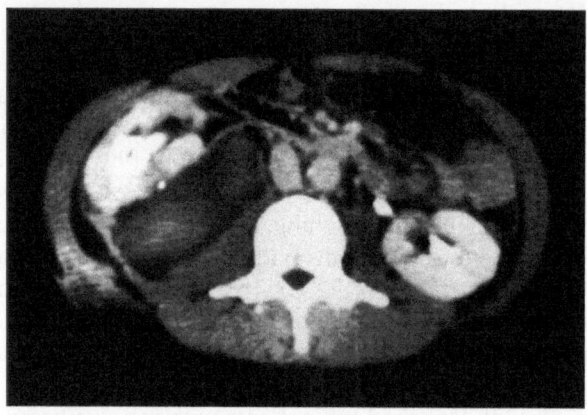

Fig. 5. CT performed 3 months after PNL in the case in Fig. 3

when the patient requires 3 or 4 units of blood after replacement of the initial blood loss (41% of their series); (3) for sudden hemorrhage more than 7 days postoperatively (35% of their series).

Perirenal hematoma caused by PNL usually subsides spontaneously (Figs. 4 and 5) without serious harm to the patient unless it is accompanied by infection. It is well known that even with needle puncture of the kidney, perirenal hematoma is observed in most cases.

Displacement of the Nephrostomy Tube

If PNL is performed as one-stage PNL, it is very difficult to reinsert the nephrostomy in the case of displacement, which may be accompanied by intractable bleeding. Therefore, it is very important to secure the nephrostomy tube, especially in obese patients.

Myocardial Infarction and Dysrhythmias

Myocardial infarction and dysrhythmias are reported in less than 1% [5] of cases, and the former has been reported in only 0.1% to 0.4% of patients [2, 3].

Late Complications

Hemorrhage

Delayed bleeding after PNL occurs in less than 1% of cases [5]. Hemorrhage due to arteriovenous fistula or pseudoaneurysm, which has been described above, may occur during this period or as late as several weeks after surgery.

Stenosis of the Urinary Tract

Injury of the ureteropelvic junction (UPJ) in PNL may cause stenosis or complete obstruction of the UPJ (Fig. 6). However, as long as the laceration is longitudinal and not circular, the operator should not worry excessively about UPJ stenosis if they use the method of endopyeloureterotomy via a transpelvic extraureteral approach. This was reported by Ono et al. [39], who incised the UPJ deep enough (1–4cm in length) to enable the operator to examine the extraureteral fat and leave a 12–14-F ureteral stent.

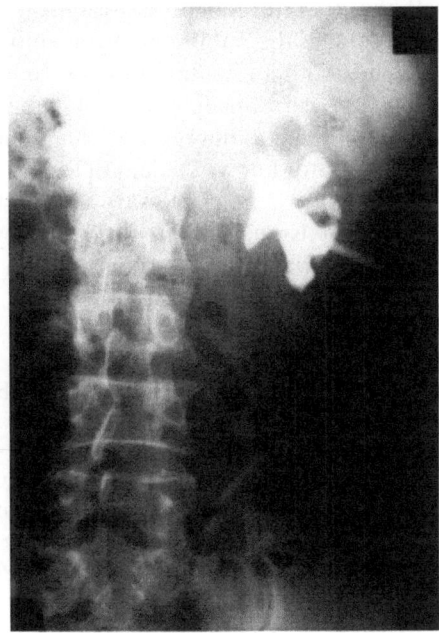

FIG. 6. Complete ureteropelvic junction obstruction on nephrostogram

Trauma of the urothelium and tissues surrounding the infundibulum results in scarring and stricture, with ultimate obliteration. Two such cases have been reported in the treatment of staghorn calculus [40].

Damage of Renal Parenchyma

Clayman et al. [5] reported that the degree of cortical loss from a 36-F percutaneous nephrostomy has been estimated to be less than 0.15% of the total renal cortical surface in experiments using pigs. Damage to renal tissue due to dilatation with a large dilator (such as 24 F) seems to be reversible or minimal, as seen on pre- and postoperative intravenous pyelography (IVP) and renal scintigrams [41]. These findings were supported by animal experiments which showed new vascular formation [17] and tissue generation [42].

Seeding of a Tumor on the Nephrostomy Tract

Seeding of a tumor on the nephrostomy tract is possible if a visually recognizable or unrecognizable tumor exists in the urinary tact. Nephrostomy tract tumor seeding following percutaneous manipulation of a ureteral carcinoma, and transitional cell carcinoma growing along an indwelling neprostomy tube track in a patient with muscle-invasive high-grade transitional cell carcinoma of the bladder, have recently been reported [43, 44].

Radiation

If the operator's hand is located under the fluoroscopy tube, i.e., if the hand appears on the TV monitor, the amount of radiation received by the operator is 120 mR with a radiation time of 2 min 8 s [45], while the limit of radiation which can be received safely by professional workers is 5000 mR per year. However, radiation due to fluoroscopy can be minimized during dilatation as follows: once the operator knows the length (depth) of the dilator to be inserted for dilatation, fluoroscopy is not necessary unless the operator feels resistance from the surrounding tissue. Radiation received by assistants such as nurses who are located 1 or 2 m away from the radiated area is negligible.

References

1. Tanahashi Y, Numata S, Chiba Y, Kanbe K, Toyoda S, Iroriya N, Kuwabara M, Orikasa S (1987) Complications of percutaneous nephrolithotomy. Kidney Dialysis 23: Suppl 206–210
2. Roth RA, Beckmann CF (1988) Complications of extracorporeal shock-wave lithotripsy and percutaneous nephrolithotomy. Urol Clin North Am 15:155–166
3. Tsuboi N, Nishimura T, Hasegawa J, Yajima I, Abe H, Kawamura N, Hirasawa S, Oki M, Sugizawa Y, Yoshida K, Akimoto M (1989) 243 cases of percutaneous nephrolithotomy. Acta Urol Jpn 35:559–563
4. Shishido S, Baba S, Ohigashi T, Muraki J, Hayashi A, Tachibana M, Deguchi N, Jitsukawa S, Hata M, Tazaki H (1990) Percutaneous removal of renal and upper

ureteral stones: clinical results and complications of 103 cases. Acta Urol Jpn 36: 997–1001

5. Clayman RV, McDougall EM, Nakada SY (1997) Endourology of the upper urinary tract: percutaneous renal and ureteral procedures. In: Walsh PC, Retik AB, Vaughan ED Jr, Wein AJ (eds) Campbell's urology. Saunders, Philadelphia, pp 2789–2874

6. Ekelund L, Lindstedt E (1990) Complications of percutaneous nephrostomy. In: Pollack HM (ed) Clinical urography. Saunders, Philadelphia, pp 2754–2760

7. Castaneda-Zuniga WR, Cardella JF (1990) Complications of percutaneous stone removal. In: Pollack HM (ed) Clinical urography. Saunders, Philadelphia, pp 2925–2933

8. Watanabe N, Mishima K, Nezu T, Tanifuji Y, Kobayashi K (1990) Sudden cardiac arrest during percutaneous nephrolithotomy under epidural anesthesia. Jpn J Anesthesiol 39:253–256

9. Cadeddu JA, Arrindell D, Moore RG (1997) Near fetal air embolism during percutaneous nephrostomy placement. J Urol 158:1519

10. Davidoff R, Bellman G (1997) Influence of technique of percutaneous tract creation on incidence of renal hemorrhage. J Urol 157:1229–1231

11. Stoller ML, Wolf JS Jr, St Lezin MA (1994) Estimated blood loss and transfusion rates associated with percutaneous nephrolithotomy. J Urol 152:1977–1981

12. Stable DP (1982) Percutaneous nephrostomy: techniques, indications, and results. Urol Clin North Am 9:15–29

13. Kessaris DN, Bellman GC, Pardalidis NP, Smith AG (1995) Management of hemorrhage after percutaneous renal surgery. J Urol 153:604–608

14. Mahaffey KG, Bolton DM, Stoller ML (1994) Urologist directed percutaneous nephrostomy tube placement. J Urol 152:1973–1976

15. Kaye KW, Clayman RV (1986) Tamponade nephrostomy catheter for percutaneous nephrostolithotomy. Urology 27:441–445

16. Cowan NC, Traill ZC, Phillips AJ, Gleeson FV (1998) Direct percutaneous transrenal embolization for renal artery injury following percutaneous nephrostomy. Br J Radiol 71:1199–1201

17. Oki M (1986) An experimental study of the operated kidney by resin injection casting in rabbits. Part 2. Post-operative renal function observing from venous cast. Jpn J Urol 77:1754–1766

18. Wolf JS (1998) Management of intraoperatively diagnosed colonic injury during percutaneous nehphrostolithotomy. Tech Urol 4:160–164

19. Daughtry JD, Rodan BA, Bean WJ (1986) Pneumocalyx following percutaneous nephrolithotomy. Urology 28:293–294

20. Gerspach JM, Bellman GC, Stoller ML, Fugelso P (1997) Conservative management of colon injury following percutaneous renal surgery. Urology 49:831–836

21. Kumar A, Kumar Banerjee G, Tewari A, Srivastava A (1994) Isolated duodenal injury during relook percutaneous nephrolithotomy. Br J Urol 74:382–383

22. Ahmed M, Reeve R (1995) Iatrogenic duodenocutaneous fistula at percutaneous nephrolithotomy managed conservatively. Br J Urol 75:416–418

23. Kondas J, Szentgyorgyi E, Vanzi L, Kiss A (1994) Splenic injury: a rare complication of percutaneous nephrolithotomy. Int Urol Nephrol 26:399–404

24. Beale TJ, Anson K, Watson M, Kellett MJ, Allen C (1997) Massive splenomegaly complicating left percutaneous renal surgery. Br J Urol 80:829–830

25. Hopper KD, Yakes WF (1990) The posterior intercostal approach for percutaneous renal procedures: risk of puncturing the lung, spleen, and liver as determined by CT. Am J Roentgenol 154:115–117

26. Reinberg Y, Moore LS, Lange PH (1989) Splenic abscess as a complication of percutaneous nephrostomy. Urology 34:274–276
27. Saxby MF (1996) Biliary peritonitis following percutaneous nephrolithotomy. Br J Urol 77:465–466
28. Kontothanassis D, Bissas A (1997) Biliary peritonitis complicating percutaneous nephrostomy. Int Urol Nephrol 29:529–531
29. Martine E, Lujan M, Paez A (1996) Puncture of the gall bladder: an unusual case of peritonitis complicating percutaneous nephrostomy. Br J Urol 77:464–465
30. Palou Redorta J, Banus Gasso JM, Prera Vilaseca A, Ramon Dalmau M, Morote Robles J, Ahmad Wahad A (1988) Renopleural fistula after percutaneous nephrolithotomy. Urol Int 43:104–106
31. Pugach JL, Moore RG, Parra RO, Steinhardt GF (1999) Massive hydrothorax and hydro-abdomen complicating percutaneous nephrolithotomy. J Urol 162:2110–2111
32. Roberts S, Bolton DM, Stoller ML (1994) Hypothermia associated with percutaneous nephrolithotomy. Urology 44:832–835
33. Charton M, Vallancien G, Veillon B, Brisset JM (1986) Urinary tract infection in percutaneous surgery for renal calculi. J Urol 135:15–17
34. Tahara H, Katoh Y, Yano H, Kanbara N, Kohri K, Kurita T (1993) Septic shock induced by extracorporeal shock wave lithotripsy treatment with percutaneous nephrostomy in 5 cases with urolithiasis. Acta Urol Jpn 39:1119–1124
35. Takeuchi H, Ueda M, Nonomura M, Hida S, Oishi K, Higashi Y, Okada Y, Kawamura J, Yoshida O (1987) Fever attack in percutaneous nephrolithotomy and transurethral ureterolithotripsy. Acta Urol Jpn 33:1357–1363
36. Nishimura T, Kawamura N, Tsuboi N, Hara M, Abe H, Akimoto M (1988) Study for relation between bacteria within stones and post-operative urinary tract infection in percutaneous nephrolithotomy. Jpn J Urol 79:283–286
37. Rao PN, Dube DA, Weightman NC, Oppenheim BA, Morris J (1991) Prediction of septicemia following endourological manipulation for stones in the upper urinary tract. J Urol 146:955–960
38. Sacha K, Szewczyk W (1996) Massive haemorrhage presenting as complication after percutaneous nephrolithotomy (PCNL). Int Urol Nephrol 28:315–318
39. Ono Y, Oshima S, Kinukawa T, Sahashi M, Yamada S (1992) Endopyelouretrotomy via a transpelvic extraureteral approach. J Urol 147:352–355
40. Weir MJ, Honey RJ (1999) Complete infundibular obliteration following percutaneous nephrolithotomy. J Urol 161:1274–1275
41. Nishimura T, Kanamori S, Abe H, Okumura S, Tsuboi N, Yoshida K, Hara M, Akimoto M (1985) Percutaneous nephrolithotomy with emphasis on large renal stones. Urology 26:143–148
42. Matsuoka K, Murakami M, Kunimi H, Ueda S, Noda S, Eto K (1988) Studies on renal damage in percutaneous nephrolithotomy: a morphological study. Jpn J Urol 79:150–154
43. Huang A, Low RK, White RV (1995) Nephrostomy tract tumor seeding following percutaneous manipulation of a ureteral carcinoma. J Urol 153:1041–1042
44. Sengupta S, Harewood L (1998) Transitional cell carcinoma growing along an indwelling nephrostomy tube track. Br J Urol 82:591
45. Nishimura T (1988) Percutaneous nephroureterolithotomy using rigid endoscope. Rinsho Hinyokika 42:215–220

Subject Index